ADULT MEN
WITH ADHD

**THE ULTIMATE GUIDE TO SOLVING ATTENTION
DEFICIT DISORDER, IMPROVING
CONCENTRATION, INCREASING
PRODUCTIVITY, ACCEPTING YOURSELF, STOP
FEELING LIKE A FAILURE, AND FINALLY
ACHIEVE SUCCESS**

By

Pansy Bradley

TABLE OF CONTENTS

INTRODUCTION

An adult may still experience ADHD, a neurological condition that first appears in childhood. Not all kids with ADHD symptoms grow up to develop the adult form of the illness, yet the prevalence of ADHD in adults is higher than once believed.

Some symptoms of childhood may fade (for example, hyperactivity) or be manifested differently later in life. Constant disorganization might lead to other negative outcomes, such as losing a job.Inattention, or trouble maintaining Focus over extended periods, is what is meant by the "attention deficit" part of attention deficit hyperactivity disorder (ADHD).

Hyperactivity in attention deficit hyperactivity disorder (ADHD) refers to sudden, difficult-to-control movement and speech. Hyperactive individuals may appear to be in constant need of motion. As a result, they make annoying noise and are seemingly always on the move.

Even though it isn't part of the official diagnostic diagnosis, impulsivity is recognized as a hallmark of this condition. Hyperactive people who are also impulsive give the impression that they act on impulse. Accidents can happen as a direct result of impulsive actions, which are typically obtrusive, impolite, and potentially harmful.

The symptoms of true ADHD are persistent and severe enough to interfere with daily life. A further need is that symptoms manifest in more than one setting. Adults with ADHD have additional challenges in the workplace and at home.ADHD is a lifelong disorder with no known treatment options, according to experts. People who suffer from this condition shouldn't lose hope, though. Various treatments can enhance one's ability to control ADHD symptoms and progress.

CHAPTER 1. UNDERSTANDING ADHD

The effects of ADHD are not limited to young people. Please find out how adult ADHD manifests itself in men and what can be done about it.

Attention deficit hyperactivity disorder (ADHD), formerly known as attention deficit disorder (ADD), can make it difficult for adults to maintain Focus and stay on task. Many individuals have ADHD, which can cause a wide range of difficulties in daily life, from personal relationships to career growth.

Problems with paying attention, being overly active, and acting impulsively are all symptoms of adult attention-deficit/hyperactivity disorder (ADHD), a mental health condition. In addition, relationship problems, poor academic or occupational performance, low self-esteem, and other issues might stem from adult ADHD.

Researchers have yet to pinpoint a single reason for ADHD, but they suspect a combination of factors, including heredity, upbringing, and unusual brain wiring, all play a role. People diagnosed with ADHD or ADD as children often continue to experience some of the disorder's symptoms as adults. Even if you weren't diagnosed with ADHD as a child, having the disorder as an adult is still possible.

In many cases, children with ADHD do not receive a diagnosis until they are adults. In the past, when knowledge of such things was far more limited, this was especially frequent. As a result, your loved ones and educators may have given you a negative name because they failed to recognize your symptoms and get to the root of the problem.

Perhaps, you may have been able to manage your ADHD symptoms as a child, only to run into difficulties when your adult responsibilities mounted. The greater the demands on your ability to organize, focus, and remain calm, the more balls you'll need to juggle in the air at once, such as a career, raising a family, and operating a household. Anyone may find this difficult, but those with ADHD may find it impossible.

No matter how hopeless things may seem, people with ADD can learn to overcome their struggles. Adults with ADHD can learn to control their condition through self-awareness, social support, and creative problem-solving. Adults with ADHD can learn to manage their symptoms and start achieving their goals at any age.

ADHD in adults is treated the same way as it is in children. Medication, psychotherapy, and the treatment of any coexisting mental health issues are all part of the standard protocol for dealing with adult ADHD.

Attention Deficit Hyperactivity Disorder In Adults: Myths & Facts

Myth: ADHD is caused by a lack of willpower. People with ADHD can zero in on tasks that pique their attention, but they may apply the same concentration level to any endeavor.

Fact: ADHD appears to be a willpower issue, but it isn't. There seems to be some chemical imbalance in the brain's control mechanisms.

Myth: People with ADHD are incapable of paying attention.

Fact: People with ADHD can often focus on tasks they enjoy. But when the work is dull or monotonous, individuals have problems concentrating no matter how hard they try.

Myth: ADHD symptoms are universal, and those with sufficient intelligence can easily overcome them.

Fact: Regardless of IQ, ADHD can affect anyone. And while everyone experiences some symptoms of ADHD from time to time, only individuals whose lives are significantly impacted regularly by these symptoms merit an ADHD diagnosis.

Myth: A person with ADHD cannot experience mental health issues like depression or anxiety.

Fact: The odds of a person with attention deficit hyperactivity disorder also suffering from another mental or learning disorder are six times higher than the average. There is often comorbidity between ADHD and other conditions.

Myth: You cannot have ADHD or ADD as an adult unless you have a childhood diagnosis.

Fact: The effects of undiagnosed ADHD can last a lifetime for many adults. They have avoided therapy because they attribute their persistent problems, such as sadness or anxiety, to untreatable underlying conditions.

Symptoms

Symptoms of ADHD may improve with age in some persons while persisting significantly in others, particularly when they reach adulthood. ADHD symptoms in adults include the inability to focus, impulsive behavior, and restlessness. The severity of the symptoms varies.

The only thing most adults with ADHD are aware of is the difficulty they sometimes have performing routine chores. Adults with ADHD may have trouble focusing and prioritizing, resulting in missed deadlines and forgotten appointments or social occasions. This lack of self-control can manifest in various ways, from mood swings and rage to impatience in traffic or long lines.

Symptoms of adult ADHD may include:

- Impulsiveness.
- Lack of order and an inability to set priorities.
- Irresponsible handling of time.
- Having trouble keeping your mind on something?
- Having difficulty switching between tasks.
- Excessive activity or unrest.
- Poor preparation.
- Lacking the ability to handle frustration well.
- Negative and positive emotions can change rapidly.
- Inability to follow through on commitments or finish projects.
- Hot temper.
- Having difficulty dealing with stress.

Differences Between Typical And ADHD Behavior

In one form or another, nearly everyone experiences symptoms that are similar to ADHD. On the other hand, you probably don't have ADHD if your problems are new or if they've only happened seldom in the past.

When symptoms of ADHD persist and interfere with significant aspects of daily life, a diagnosis is made. These bothersome symptoms have their origins in childhood and remain throughout adulthood.

Some symptoms of ADHD are similar to those of other illnesses, such as anxiety and mood disorders, making diagnosis challenging in adults. In addition, many grown-ups diagnosed with ADHD also struggle with another form of mental illness.

Causes

However, studies are still being conducted to determine what causes ADHD. Possible contributors to the onset of attention deficit hyperactivity disorder are:

- **Genetics**. Research suggests that genetics may contribute to the emergence of attention deficit hyperactivity disorder (ADHD).

- **Environment**. Exposure to lead during childhood is one potential environmental risk factor.

- **Developmental issues**. Possible contributors include central nervous system issues at critical ages.

Effects Of Adult ADHD

Adults who only now realize they have attention deficit hyperactivity disorder (ADHD) often experienced the negative effects of this condition for quite some time. It's understandable if you've been feeling like you're treading water lately, what with all the pressure that comes from putting things off until the last minute or being unprepared for what has to be done.

Perhaps you've come to view yourself negatively after hearing people call you names like "lazy," "irresponsible," or "dumb" because of your forgetfulness or inability to finish certain duties.

Untreated and undiagnosed ADHD can have far-reaching consequences and disrupt many facets of a person's life.

- **Physical and mental health problems**

Compulsive eating, substance misuse, anxiety, chronic stress and tension, and low self-esteem are just some of the health issues that ADHD symptoms can exacerbate. In addition, neglecting essential checkups, missing doctor's appointments, disregarding medical instructions, and missing drug doses can all lead to serious complications.

- **Stress from work and a lack of funds**

Adults with ADHD frequently struggle in their chosen profession and suffer from a profound sense of unfulfillment. Maintaining employment, adhering to company policies, completing tasks on time, and sticking to a 9-to-5 schedule may all be challenging. In addition, unpaid bills, misplaced documents, late fines, and debt brought on by careless spending are all signs of financial mismanagement.

- **Relationship issues**

Adhd symptoms might disrupt your professional, personal, and family life. There's a good chance you're sick of hearing your loved ones tell you to clean up, pay attention, and get your life in order. On the other hand, your loved ones may be wounded and angry by your "irresponsibility" or "insensitivity," as these words are used by others who are not close to you.

Disgrace, frustration, hopelessness, disappointment, and a lack of self-esteem are only some of the negative outcomes of ADHD. For example, you may feel hopeless that you'll never be able to get your life together and achieve your goals.

Many adults find learning they have attention deficit hyperactivity disorder reassuring and encouraging development. It lets you finally comprehend your situation and realize that you are not at fault. Your struggles are not due to a lack of willpower or a defect in your character; they are the outcome of attention deficit hyperactivity disorder.

Working Around Adult ADHD

Thinking something is fundamentally wrong with you is a common outcome of living with Attention Deficit Hyperactivity Disorder. Being unique is acceptable, though. ADHD is not responsible for a person's mental or physical abilities. Even if you might have more trouble in some situations, you can still find your niche and be successful. Knowing and playing to your talents is essential.

It may assist in viewing ADD as a personality profile, like any other, consisting of positive and bad characteristics. ADHD symptoms, such as impulsivity and disorganization, are not always accompanied by a lack of creativity, passion, energy, or creative ideas. First, you need to identify your strengths, and then you can create a setting that plays to those.

Self-help For Adult ADHD

With an awareness of the difficulties posed by ADHD and the aid of systematic approaches, positive improvements can be made in one's life. Many adults with ADD/ADHD have learned effective strategies for coping with their condition, capitalizing on their strengths, and leading full and rewarding lives.

You probably won't need help from anyone else, at least not right immediately. However, you can help yourself a great deal and bring your symptoms under control by doing some of the things listed below.

- **Get some exercise and try to eat well**

Get plenty of intense exercises regularly; it's great for relieving stress and anxiety and channeling negative emotions. To reduce emotional swings, consume a varied diet high in nutrients and low in sugary foods.

- **Get a good night's rest**

Focus, stress management, productivity, and staying on top of your duties are already challenging enough without being overly sleep deprived. Try to sleep for 7–9 hours every night, and put down the phone an hour before bed.

- **Learn to manage your time more effectively**

Giving yourself deadlines for everything, even the smallest chores, is important. Set alarms and timers to keep yourself on track. Add frequent rest periods within your schedule.

If you take care of things as they come in, you won't have to worry about falling behind or avoiding the work. Instead, you should prioritize time-sensitive jobs and record all instructions, messages, and insights in writing.

- **Improve your relationships**

Organize get-togethers with your pals and show up on time for them. Maintain in-person and online vigilance; pay attention when others are talking, and avoid rushing your communications. Connect with others who will sympathize with and support you through your ADHD challenges.

- **Make sure your office is a positive place to work**

Use tools like lists, color coding, reminders, notes to self, rituals, and files to keep yourself organized. Do something that excites and fascinates you if at all possible. Take note of when you are most productive, and try replicating that setting at work. Working in tandem with others who are less creative but more organized can be useful.

- **Practice mindfulness**

Frequent mindfulness meditation can assist you in calming your busy mind and improving your emotional control, even though it may be challenging for some people with ADHD even to consider it. Start with a short meditation session and gradually lengthen it as your practice improves.

- **Don't take the blame; ADHD is to blame**

Adults with ADHD often have a negative self-perception or blame themselves for their difficulties. Depression, anxiety, and low self-esteem are all possible outcomes of this. If you've been diagnosed with ADHD and have a certain brain structure, it may be impossible to change either. However, you can learn to live with these limitations and even thrive despite them.

Coexisting conditions

Even though ADHD is not the root cause of any mental or developmental issues, it frequently co-occurs with other diseases, making treatment more difficult. The following are some of them:

- **Mood disorders**. Depression, bipolar disorder, and other mood disorders are common among individuals with ADHD. Even if ADHD isn't directly linked to mood disorders, a history of setbacks and frustrations at the hands of the disorder can amplify the effects of depression.
- **Anxiety disorders**. ADHD adults are at a higher risk for developing anxiety disorders. Extreme worrying, agitation, and other uncomfortable feelings are possible side effects of anxiety disorders. In addition, the difficulties and disappointments arising from ADHD might amplify any pre-existing anxiety.

- **Other psychiatric disorders**. Adults diagnosed with ADHD are at increased risk for related mental health issues.

- **Learning disabilities**. Compared to what would be predicted, considering their age, IQ, and education, adults with ADHD may do worse on academic tests. Difficulties in both comprehension and expression are common among those with learning disabilities.

When An Adult Needs Outside Assistance For ADHD

After trying to control your ADHD symptoms on your own and still finding that they are causing problems in your daily life, professional treatment may be the next logical step. Medications, self-help groups, individual therapy, career counseling, educational support, and more all aid adults with ADHD.

Adults with ADD should be treated by a multidisciplinary team that includes the patient's primary care physician, psychiatrist, psychologist, therapist, and even the patient's family and spouse, just as they would be for a child.
Experts in attention deficit hyperactivity disorder (ADHD) can teach you how to control your emotions and impulses, organize your life, increase productivity at work and home, calm your temper, and have more effective conversations.

Having ADHD Does Not Automatically Make One Hyperactive

Hyperactivity is a symptom of ADHD that is far less common in adults than children and teenagers. Hyperactivity is only a noticeable symptom in a minority of individuals with ADHD. Remember that despite what the term may imply, hyperactivity is not a necessary criterion for a diagnosis of attention deficit hyperactivity disorder (ADHD).

CHAPTER 2. CAUSES OF ADHD

The specific origins of ADHD remain a medical mystery. The symptoms and the underlying causes of ADHD in children and adults are contingent on many factors.

Nearly 3 out of every 100 American people are believed to have attention deficit hyperactivity disorder. But unfortunately, many people may live with the disorder without realizing it. Below are a few causes of ADHD in adult men:

Genetics

In most situations, it is believed that the genes you receive from your parents are a crucial component in developing ADHD. The prevalence of ADHD runs in families, with studies showing that both parents and children of an ADHD patient share the disorder at higher rates. Nevertheless, it is unlikely that a single genetic flaw is responsible for ADHD. Instead, the inheritance of the disorder is assumed to be more complex.

Brain Function And Structure

Researchers have found some potential abnormalities in the brains of those with ADHD and those without the disorder, but the relevance of these findings is still unclear. Brain scans, for instance, have revealed that ADHD patients can have abnormally large or tiny brain regions.

Other research has pointed to a possible dysfunction or imbalance of neurotransmitters in the brains of patients with ADHD.

Consequently, the following are among the most common triggers of ADHD in adult men:

- Genetics.
- Lack of proper prenatal nourishment.
- Prenatal substance abuse includes both alcohol and drug use.
- Premature birth.
- Congenital brain damage.
- Malnutrition in young children
- Simultaneous mental health conditions.

Some of the reasons why ADHD manifests itself in adolescents and adults include:

- Brain injury.
- Environmental exposure to toxins.
- Constant and excessive consumption of alcohol.

Adult ADHD Risk Factors

Adults with either early-onset or late-onset forms of ADHD may also deal with various other health issues. They may contribute to the development of ADHD or be precursors to the disorder. The following other medical disorders, behavioral problems, and lifestyle choices may be related to ADHD:

- Poor nutrition.
- Lack of exercise.
- Having obesity.
- Cannabis dependence.
- Alcohol dependence.
- Substance use.
- Generalized anxiety disorder.
- Depression.
- Sleep disorders.
- Learning disorders.
- Personality disorders.
- Conduct disorders.
- Autism spectrum disorders.

Too much time spent on social media has been linked in one 2018 study to an increase in ADHD symptoms in young adults.

Nine symptoms of inattention, such as problems with organization and task completion, and nine symptoms of hyperactivity and impulsivity, such as problems with Focus and staying on target, were reported by students themselves.

Teens were classed as having ADHD symptoms if they reported six or more symptoms across both categories.

To anyone who has ever scrolled through their feed absentmindedly (and let's be honest, who hasn't), this may come as no surprise. But more research is needed to establish the nature of the relationship between adult ADHD and social media use.

CHAPTER 3. HOW I KNOW I HAVE ADULT ADHD (SYMPTOMS)

You are never punctual. An event is utterly forgotten if it is not entered into your calendar. What about the tasks you have been avoiding? You tend to get your best work done the night before a deadline, so even though they are stacking up quickly, you shouldn't worry.

You may feel as though you've developed these traits over time. But since you can't change who you are, why try? Stay the same.

However, if these traits interfere with your personal and professional life, you may be experiencing adult attention-deficit/hyperactivity disorder (ADHD).

As opposed to children, it is far more difficult to recognize the symptoms of ADHD in an adult. Michael Manos, Ph.D., a pediatric behavioral health specialist, teaches how to recognize and deal with adult ADHD symptoms and determine if these issues warrant professional help.

Adult ADHD Symptoms

Consider your life and your decisions; if you've left a trail of "incompletions," as Dr. Manos calls them (unfinished job, unfinished school work, missing dates, forgotten anniversaries), you may be dealing with attention deficit hyperactivity disorder.

"Adults with ADHD tend to abandon projects midway through," Dr. Manos explains. For an adult with ADHD, these incomplete tasks are the main functional trait that causes problems.

ADHD is diagnosed via a three-stage approach. Among other things, a doctor diagnosing adult ADHD will check for the following:

ADHD symptoms are detrimental to a person's life.
Possible environmental influences on the exhibited behavior.
Another mental disorder is present.

If you don't have dysfunction, then you don't have a problem, explains Dr. Manos.

"When people have serious problems in their lives, such as not being able to pay the rent or send a child to the school they desire, or when someone close to them has died or gone through a traumatic event, those problems may be distracting them, causing them to forget things or become irritated or forgetful, or even to exhibit symptoms of attention deficit hyperactivity disorder."

Approximately 4.4% of American adults and 2.5% of adults globally are diagnosed with ADHD. Fifty-plus percent of people with ADHD also have other mental health issues, such as depression or anxiety. One study from 2019 found that the rate of increase in ADHD diagnoses among adults was four times that among children.

Without treatment for ADHD in adults, either through counseling or medication, "the adult leaves a trail of incompletions in their path," says Dr. Manos, which can cause anxiety and depression. Most people with ADHD can also be diagnosed with a depressive or anxiety disorder.

To treat adult ADHD effectively, making a correct diagnosis and uncovering any contributing factors is crucial. There are 18 symptoms used to diagnose attention deficit hyperactivity disorder (9 inattentive and 9 hyperactivity).

A child must display six symptoms in two or more situations before an ADHD diagnosis can be made (like at home and school). Adults need to demonstrate five or more of these in any setting.

Inattentive Symptoms Of Adult ADHD

The Focus, in this case, is of two types:

When we focus on what we already care about—our interests, knowledge, and desires—we engage in automatic attention. So, for example, on a nice day, you might feel compelled to go outside and enjoy the sunshine and fresh air.

Focusing intently on anything necessitates what's known as "directed attention" or "effortful attention." Therefore, even though the weather is nice, you concentrate on the job rather than enjoying the sunshine. You'll need serious self-discipline and focus on completing the work at hand.

Everyone uses both types of attention, but problems arise when one's capacity to control, sustain, and return Focus is compromised.

Dr. Manos explains that those with ADHD have "impaired directed attention." "They are unable to apply effortful attention. Instead, they actively shun it in favor of automatic attention tasks.

1. Inattentive to details

Although it may seem obvious, one of the telltale signs of attention deficit hyperactivity disorder is difficulty focusing and remembering details. For example, perhaps your partner informed you that the rear door's extra key was stored in the nightstand's top right drawer, but you went to the wrong one.

Or you may have rushed through a presentation and forgotten some important details. You may use some assistance in paying closer attention to your immediate environment.

2. Having trouble staying on task

Perhaps because you have so much on your plate, you tend to jump about from one task to another. You've always boasted about your ability to juggle multiple tasks at once, after all. But if you're feeling overwhelmed because you have six unfinished projects, assignments, or activities and know you need to accomplish something, this could be an issue.

3. Trouble listening

You look completely disinterested when someone tries to have a one-on-one conversation with you. But, of course, you're not deliberately ignoring them; perhaps an idea came to mind that made you think of a funny story, and the next thing you know, your mind is somewhere else, waiting for a chance to express itself.

It could be your ADHD acting up if anyone has said you don't pay attention in class or that you seem to zone out when discussing.

4. A lack of commitment

Not only do you forget key dates like birthdays and anniversaries, but you also have difficulty keeping your word and getting things done when they need to. When other people criticize you, it could be challenging to articulate exactly what went wrong with your decision-making skills. But, ultimately, you meant well.You may have every intention of following through, but as Dr. Manos points out, sometimes we don't. So you choose to ignore it instead.

5. Disorganization

Having a lack of organization can manifest itself in many forms. For example, dishes may end up in the wrong cupboard, while bright green shirts may end up in the whites-only laundry. In addition, having a disorganized home may give the impression that you can't find what you need when you need it or may make you feel frustrated and frazzled.

However you choose to frame it, when your method of organizing stands between you and your goals of getting things done on time and experiencing a sense of accomplishment, it is time to reevaluate.

6. Procrastination

Do memories of staying late to finish a paper the night before it was due to make you smile? Even though you no longer have the luxury of procrastinating as you did in high school, procrastination can still serve you well in several other contexts.

There's a chance you may not even notice them at first. The Friendsgiving you're organizing is coming up, but you haven't gotten around to responding to texts, returning phone calls, or creating a Facebook event. Perhaps you've overused the snooze button on your alarm clock and regretted the extra sleep you've gained at the expense of getting up and preparing for work.

Dr. Manos defines procrastination as the avoidance of having to apply effortful attention. Adults with ADHD are more likely to put off tasks they don't want to undertake in favor of easy ones.

7. Often misplaces stuff

You always seem to forget where you put your phone or car keys as you leave a room, and then you spend the next hour searching fruitlessly for them. In addition, because of your disorganized nature, you frequently lose track of important items, such as assignments or work projects.

8. Prone to distraction

In the same way that a dog is attracted to a bright new toy, you find yourself quickly distracted. Something happening outside the window might easily derail a conversation in the middle of it.

Alternatively, perhaps you check your phone during a meeting and realize half an hour has passed since you were so preoccupied with whatever was on it. If you're so preoccupied with something else that it's clear to everyone around you, it can give you severe anxiety.

9. Forgetfulness

Nothing is safe from being forgotten; dates, cooking times, and other reminders are all tossed to the wind. So it's not horrible if you repeat the same story twice or thrice without realizing you've already told it.

However, you may come across as uncaring or inattentive to the requirements of your friends, family, boss, or significant other if you forget key things that they have shared with you.

"At some point in their lives, everyone suffers from a lack of Focus. Dr. Manos asserts that it is human nature to misplace or lose things frequently. It's not that these actions are what cause ADHD in adulthood. However, adults with ADHD have a problem since they frequently engage in these behaviors.

Hyperactivity Symptoms Of Adult ADHD

It is much simpler to identify hyperactivity in kids than in adults. For example, a hyperactive child may become overtly disruptive, restless, and anxious when placed in a structured setting like a classroom. However, adults with ADHD may always give the impression that they are rushing or are overburdened by their workload simply because they have taken on too much.

Dr. Manos explains that adults' hyperactive tendencies "manifest" in different ways.

What I mean is this:

1. Fidgeting

Whether it's doodling, taking notes, or fumbling with your phone, it's not productive to be restless in a meeting. Fidgeting can manifest itself in various ways, including the compulsion to bite nails or tap your feet.

2. Frequent standing up from your chair

Perhaps you have trouble sitting still for long periods, so you plan many breaks throughout the day to get up and move around, only to realize that you've spent much of that time engaged in something other than the work at hand. Unless these brief bursts of movement interfere with your productivity, there's no reason to worry.

3. Chronic restlessness

Chronic restlessness symptoms include fidgeting and needing to get up and move about the room constantly. In addition to being unable to focus during work hours, you also have trouble sleeping at times when you need to.

Have you ever gotten out of bed or delayed going to sleep because you felt like you needed to get things done, even if you knew you could wait until the morning? Your inability to settle down and get any work done may be a symptom of attention deficit hyperactivity disorder (ADHD).

4. Having a hard time focusing on quiet tasks

If you have problems sitting still, you may find it difficult to engage in solitary activities like reading a book, meditating, or watching a full-length film without becoming distracted or spoiling the experience for yourself or others. Likewise, you may find it hard to sleep unless you have something on in the background to divert your attention from your racing thoughts, such as a movie or music. Dr. Manos adds that sometimes people can't even sit through an interesting movie.

5. You're always on-the-go

You've got a lot of peps and a can-do attitude in your step. You can juggle multiple tasks at once and never seem to slow down. However, every one of your waking hours is occupied with something different, and even when you're trying to get anything done, you find yourself being sidetracked.

If you're a person who's always moving forward with life and can multitask easily, this may not be a problem. However, Dr. Manos claims that hyperactive people are extremely productive.

Adults with attention deficit hyperactivity disorder frequently take on more responsibilities than they can handle. As a result, they don't always finish what they start, and they often don't finish the extra work they've accumulated for themselves.

6. Talking too much

You might be familiar with the adage "mind over matter." Particularly when you have an idea you have to share with the world; when sharing a story, your impulsivity often takes over, or you may feel compelled to overshare personal information because you "had to get it out of your system."

7. Interrupting others or completing their statements

You tend to jump to the point and act almost on impulse in a conversation. You probably are, even if you don't mean to interrupt someone while they're talking. When that occurs, you inadvertently quicken the pace to keep things flowing at your rate of preference.

8 Difficulty with line-waiting

You become angry and impatient in long queues, whether at the supermarket checkout or in bumper-to-bumper traffic on the highway. To a significant extent, this stems from the chronic restlessness that sets up whenever the pace of life around you slows down.

9. Interrupting or bothering other people

Hyperactivity can cause your thoughts and actions to move at a breakneck pace, making it difficult to keep other people's personal space in mind. It could be that you never knock before entering a room, offer your opinion when it isn't asked for, or insist on always having the final say in a debate.

It's easy to write off impulsive behaviors as a natural part of your personality, but if they're wreaking havoc in your social life, it might be time to get tested for ADHD.

CHAPTER 4. CHALLENGES OF PEOPLE WITH ADULT ADHD

According to the National Survey on Mental Health and Wellbeing in Australia, 11% of children and adolescents met the signs and symptoms of ADHD. However, if half of those with ADHD continue to show symptoms into adulthood, then as many as 5 percent of Australian adults may be affected.

Evidence from overseas suggests that the true figure is closer to 3–4% of people who still have symptoms of ADHD. For example, 8 and 9 million adults in the United States are coping with the effects of ADHD.

Suppose the number is 3% or 5%. In that case, it is obvious that a sizable proportion of Australian adults are still dealing with ADHD into adulthood and that many have not been diagnosed or are not getting the therapy they need. Adults with ADHD face challenges in their personal and professional lives due to their condition's symptoms. However, even having ADHD, no one is exempt from the consequences of their actions.Although you or a loved one facing the challenges of ADHD may feel helpless, effective treatments are available. Make an appointment with a doctor to obtain a thorough diagnosis so you can manage your ADHD as an adult and resume living the life you want.

For a better understanding of why it is crucial to recognize the disease, get a good diagnosis made, and, most importantly, treat it, let's examine the top 10 challenges experienced by adults with ADHD:

1. Maintaining Focus

Adults with ADHD frequently struggle with inattention or the inability to focus on a single task at any time. As a result, adults with ADHD may be more easily distracted and have a harder time maintaining Focus. Not only are children but also adults with ADHD highly susceptible to distractions such as movement, conversations occurring outside of their office, and the blare of the radio or television.

2. Punctuality

Is it hard for you to keep to a schedule? Adults with ADHD have a particularly difficult time managing their time. They are chronically late for everything from work to picking up their kids from school to important meetings. People with ADHD have a much higher propensity for missing deadlines than the general population.

3. Staying Organized
Most ADHD adults struggle to track time or prioritize tasks regularly at work. Organizing, prioritizing, and devoting sufficient time and energy to completing all duties and paying attention to the details makes paperwork particularly troublesome. As a result, adults with ADHD often find it difficult to keep thorough records, locate critical documents, and submit reports on time.

4. Safe Driving
The assistance of a doctor is needed right away for this challenge. Findings suggest that compared to people without ADHD, those with the disorder are at approximately 50% higher risk of being involved in fatal car accidents
Adults with ADHD often struggle with inattentiveness and distraction, which can compromise driving safety. Some adults with ADHD claim that listening to music while Driving helps them concentrate.

5. Completing Projects
Having trouble finishing whatever you start? Sound familiar? People with ADHD often struggle to complete projects, which can negatively affect their professional and personal lives. It's common practice to get 90% through a project before moving on to something else. Adults with ADHD may be jacks of all trades but masters of none because they constantly switch gears and start new pursuits.

6. Sleeping Enough
Most people have trouble sleeping because they have too much on their minds, even if this isn't a recognized medical condition. Adults with ADHD often struggle with sleep deprivation. Fifty percent of kids and eighty percent of adults with ADHD have trouble falling asleep, staying asleep, getting quality sleep, and waking up refreshed, per ADDitude magazine.

7. Maintaining One Job
Adults with ADD/ADHD have much more difficulty maintaining employment than their typically healthy peers. Finding and keeping a job can be challenging for people with ADHD because of symptoms including impulsivity and hyperactivity. In contrast to the 72% of persons without ADHD who could do so in the same poll, just 50% of those with ADHD could maintain full-time employment.

8. Committing Names, Duties, And Deadlines To Memory
Adults with ADHD often have trouble remembering things, which can cause personal, work, and home problems. For example, they often have trouble remembering things like names, where they put things when they need to see the doctor, and other significant dates and events.

9. Experiencing Boredom Easily
Adults with ADHD face a particularly formidable foe in the workplace: boredom. This is true even for those who have found a way to make a living doing what they love. It doesn't take long for them to lose interest in a new skill they've learned. But on the other hand, they always look for anything new and exciting and thrive when given new tasks and responsibilities.

10. Developing Relationships With Others
Even the most common ADHD symptoms can negatively impact maintaining balance in interpersonal relationships. Adults with ADHD may have trouble focusing and delegating tasks, making them poor team members and partners. This person is typically rude, has trouble listening, and is quick to lose their temper.

Although these challenges may appear overwhelming, several effective treatments exist for individuals with ADHD. ADHD treatment used to center around kids. There are more options accessible now because more adults are admitting they have problems and looking for help.

Getting an accurate diagnosis from a medical practitioner is very important for you or a loved one dealing with ADHD.

CHAPTER 5. THE REALITY OF ADHD IN MEN

Our understanding of the challenges specific to women with ADHD has greatly improved. How about the condition of men, who comprise the other half of the population? Relationship success requires an awareness of the stresses and routines under which a man functions after obtaining a diagnosis.

After spending more than a decade helping couples in which at least one member has ADHD or ADD, I've discovered some commonalities between the lives of men with ADHD and the women who love them.

I am not generalizing about all men. What is written here is not meant to be taken as advice for every man with ADHD. Women are not immune to these patterns. However, consider whether any of the following five characteristics ring true while you reflect on your partner.

1. Embarrassment About ADHD And The Workplace

ADHD adults often experience issues at work, such as conflicts with coworkers, dissatisfaction with the work environment, boredom at work, disciplinary action, and even termination.

Work is a major aspect of many men's identities. They feel humiliated and extremely downhearted because of their employment problems. Low self-esteem and ADHD symptoms can make it difficult for men to maintain employment, even when they excel at work.

Client: "I was more afraid of being evaluated for my work because I had no idea whether I was doing a good or bad job." Many men say they put in extra hours at work to remain on top of everything and get things done—several types of stress-strain relationships.

Men who struggle at work because of ADHD often do so in silence out of fear of social stigma. For example, a coworker of mine was fired from three successive executive roles because he couldn't keep up with the paperwork. After the third defeat, he was too ashamed to see his wife again, so he started leaving the house and "working" instead of staying in bed.

In other cases, the partners of men with ADHD make the difficulties they face in the workplace and the possibility of losing their jobs worse. Adults with ADHD, for instance, struggle to begin the job search process because of the sheer volume of information available. Planning, effort, and persistence are necessary for a search, as is the ability to take rejection gracefully. These qualities do not typically characterize symptoms of ADHD. Adding stress and criticism to the search process is not helpful for the person with ADHD and their partner.

Instead of addressing their feelings about finding jobs, I've witnessed men refuse to look for one. Recently I heard from a man who said, "I feel fear about seeking a job, so I become stubborn." Many men view fear and tension as signs of weakness; therefore, acting steadfastly, even when doing so is counterproductive, is a way to feel more powerful.

Advice For Men With ADHD

- Engage the services of a competent ADHD coach to assist you in mastering the dull but essential aspects of your work.

- Conflict with coworkers and disruptive conduct are two of the most significant challenges employees with ADHD face on the job. Therefore, you should make your difficulty controlling your anger a primary focus of your treatment.

- Set small, achievable goals. This will help you feel less overwhelmed and keep you going.

Advice For Partners Of Men With ADHD

- Stop worrying and give yourself a break from the stress of applying for jobs. Instead, it would help if you encouraged them to seek professional help from a recruiter or an employment agency.

- Avoid adding to the humiliation of being fired or having issues at work. Instead, remember the challenges people with ADHD face when trying to maintain or secure employment, and keep an open mind. This may help your partner feel more comfortable seeking assistance.

- Encourage partners with ADHD to control their emotional impulsivity.

- For a significant portion of your life together, you will likely have to shoulder the financial responsibilities of supporting the other.

2. Difficulties In Managing Emotions, Particularly For ADD Men

One of the hallmarks of attention deficit hyperactivity disorder is emotional dysregulation or an overreaction to stimuli. In my experience, guys are more likely to have problems controlling their anger than women. Angry men are tolerated in our culture, while angry women face much backlash.

Men with ADHD are less likely to recognize their emotional difficulties. Many men will legitimately use anger to get their partners to back off and then blame their partners for their rage.

"You initiated this disagreement; therefore, I snapped at you," the husband said to his wife. So what? Could you give it up and move on? Another person yelling and being disrespectful to his partner denied that he was angry. Another person who often inflicted pain and suffering with his outbursts told me, "Everything is OK because I've been used to going from zero to sixty in a split second."

Advice For Men With ADHD

- Recognize the true nature of your anger management problems: Negative effects of ADHD on personal and professional life. Help is required for them. To help stabilize your mood, you may take medication, learn mindfulness techniques, or start exercising more.

- Please seek professional help to identify the causes of your emotional outbursts and learn how to manage them.

Advice For Partners Of Men With ADHD

- Distinguish the person with ADHD from the disorder itself. This is a symptom, not a character flaw. Instead of reacting aggressively, telling him how his anger affects you would be better.

- With the help of your partner, establish verbal cues to end disagreements before they escalate. For example, when I see my spouse becoming worked up but not realizing it, we have an "aardvark" agreement. The message conveyed by this particular term is "silence," that is, "take a deep breath and relax." We've had great success with it.

3. Retreat As A Method Of Managing ADHD In Men

According to research, men struggle more than women to heal from conflict. After an argument, individuals have a harder time relaxing, and their blood pressure stays elevated for longer. Most men want to avoid conflicts because of the negative physiological effects they have on them.

Often, men who have ADHD report feeling that they are always being criticized for their lack of progress at home and in the workplace. Many men avoid conflict because they can't become reliable due to distractions and planning issues. As a result, you can resort to deceptive practices like lying and withdrawing emotionally.

The retreat is seen as beneficial and essential by some. He said, "It is easier to silently commit myself to conduct measures that will make up for them" rather than constantly disagree with his wife, so he covers up his faults. Because connection and trust are crucial to long-lasting relationships, it's important to comprehend male avoidance to combat it.

Advice For Men With ADHD

- Contemplate the benefits you receive from retreating (lower levels of immediate discomfort) and the drawbacks you risk (a good relationship). Then, recognize the hurt you've caused your loved ones by using avoidance or isolation as a coping mechanism. Realizing that your isolation is to blame is the first step toward fixing the problem.
- Try brainstorming new ways to talk with your partner (and maybe a therapist) about painful memories and events.

Verbal clues, planning emotional dialogues ahead of time rather than having them on the spur of the moment, and practicing awareness when criticizing oneself are all possibilities.

- Resist the urge to retreat. Taking positive action to strengthen your relationship is your only option. Look into "learning conversations" and other forms of communication that might keep you involved without escalating into a heated argument.

Advice For Partners Of Men With ADHD

- Recognize that you are a critic and adjust your approach accordingly. Talk to your ADHD partner gently at first, ask for what you want rather than telling them what to do, and remember that they have a right to their opinion regardless of whether you agree with it.

- Please do not create a situation where your partner believes he can never satisfy you.

4. Men With ADHD Have Trouble Expressing Their Feelings

Generally, we don't do a very good job teaching our young men and boys healthy ways to deal with their feelings and emotions. We instead instill in them the values of toughness, stoicism, and silence. The fact that men with ADHD have trouble picking up on the feelings of those around them doesn't help matters.
Understanding and expressing one's feelings is a skill that requires time, effort, and, for some, bravery to master. For this reason, males need to work on becoming aware of and expressing their emotions as part of their therapy.

Adults might refer to a list of "I-focused" emotion words while having dialogues about their feelings. Feelings can be discussed with more nuance after using them. Getting some practice is important when things aren't quite as intense.

Advice For Men With ADHD

- To reinforce emotional words, create multiple daily reminders for a full month. For example, you should ask yourself, "How am I feeling right now?" for a full minute when your alarm goes off. Then, if you need more time to practice, you can do it again for another month. As time goes on, you'll get better at naming and articulating your emotions.

Advice For Partners Of Men With ADHD

- It may be easier for women to open up about their feelings than for men. Inspire the man you care about to hone his abilities in this area. Also, don't try to guess how he'll react. If your partner doesn't react emotionally as you had intended or say what you would have said, your disappointment will send the message that they are a failure.

5. Reluctance To Accept The ADHD Diagnosis

The vast majority of the female patients I see and speak with have come to terms with their ADHD diagnosis. They see introspection and self-criticism as healthy practices that lead to growth. On the other hand, many men appear to dismiss ADHD as a real disorder.

They fear that if they admit they have ADHD, others will start blaming them for the difficulties in their relationships. One man said, "For a while now, she has been entirely focused on me as the problem in our relationship." The act of "admitting" to having ADHD would lend credence to this attribution.

However, it's not a one-way street. A common pattern among men who have ADHD is to place the blame for relationship problems on their partners who do not have the disorder.

Partners who don't also struggle with ADHD are portrayed as hostile and irritated by their actions. Instead of facing the potential emotional turmoil of an ADHD diagnosis, it's easier to blame the partner who doesn't have the disorder.

- If you and your partner both have ADHD, it doesn't matter what you call it. So get evaluated. The doors to numerous life-improving therapy alternatives may be thrown open.

- If you're worried about being blamed for any problems in the relationship in the event of a diagnosis, it's important to talk about it with your partner and figure out what you can do to fix things.

Advice For Partners Of Men With ADHD

- Put an end to the ADHD blame game. Both the ADHD symptoms themselves and your reactions to them might cause problems. There's work for you and your partner to undertake. Men are more likely to get evaluated if their partners admit they have problems, too.

Positively Engage Your Man In These 8 Ways

- Start talking gently rather than aggressively.

- If your partner isn't looking at you, wait for him to switch his attention to you before carrying on.

- Maintain your decorum even though you're fuming inside.

- Try explaining your problems using "I" statements rather than "you" comments that blame someone else.

- Stay away from nagging and judging.

- Decide not to add to your partner's embarrassment.

- To the extent possible, hold hands or otherwise engage in physical contact.

- Acknowledge the good things that happen to you and make it a practice to see the humor in difficult circumstances.

CHAPTER 6. THE COMMON MISCONCEPTIONS ABOUT ADHD

People continue to hold numerous incorrect notions and even spread certain blatant myths, concerning ADHD, despite revolutionary research and unequivocal neurological discoveries that disprove these ideas. Here, you will find evidence-based facts on attention deficit hyperactivity disorder.

ADHD Myth #1: It is usually a disorder and a disability.

Here, we're bucking the trend. ADHD is an umbrella term for a group of symptoms. DSM-5, released by the American Psychiatric Association, classifies it as a mental disorder. So psychiatrists, psychiatrists, and other medical professionals can confirm that this is a disorder.

OK, fine. However, the phrase "disorder" has a connotation of negativity and ignores the many admirable qualities that people with ADHD possess.

Is it a mental disorder to have high empathy, creativity, and energy levels? Is it a disorder to have an instantaneous intuitive understanding of virtually everything you encounter? Is it a disorder to be very discerning and inquisitive?

We agree that ADHD is best understood as a "context disorder." However, there are times when this becomes a problem.
According to ADHD specialist Thom Hartmann, "if a left-handed individual has a job cutting origami with right-handed scissors, that does not mean they have a handicap; they have a context issue." Likewise, there is a context disorder if a short person tries to play basketball.

In many institutional and professional settings, ADHD can also be viewed as a disability. Extra time to finish projects and a clutter-free work environment are examples of reasonable adjustments that people with ADHD are entitled to.

Everything has its place and time, but generally, viewing ADHD as a disorder or a disability is detrimental to your personal growth.

Those who have ADHD are not defective, disabled, ill, or abnormal in any way. We were only made in different molds.

Also, there is no surefire diagnostic test for ADHD, so don't assume you have it if you think you might. The medical establishment tends towards an "all-or-none" model, where a person either has a psychiatric condition or does not. The truth is that personality quirks and mental illness are too intertwined to be disentangled.

Can you be described as "very active" or "hyperactive"? Do you think quickly and imaginatively, or are you easily distracted? No simple blood test can reveal the answers to these queries. Instead, each person expresses their features in various ways that make up a complicated continuum or spectrum.

According to psychiatrist David Rettew, MD, there may be some value in adopting a more nuanced perspective of psychiatric disorders that recognizes the connections between these conditions and a person's temperament and character. One advantage of this perspective is that it may be less judgmental.

Reminding someone that "everyone lives on this spectrum someplace and that he is somewhere at the top but that he can lower that level down with little intervention and hard work" is often more comforting than simply telling them, "You 'have' ADHD."

ADHD Myth #2: ADHD isn't real.

A very real distinction in neurobiology is ADHD. There are chemical changes in the brain's management systems of persons who live with the symptoms of ADHD, according to extensive scientific studies. SPECT, FMRI, and CT scans, among others, have provided hard evidence that our brains are "wired" in distinctive ways.

The details of impaired executive functioning, susceptibility to dopamine-seeking cycles, and so on will not be discussed further here. However, there is a fundamental biological basis for differences in abilities to focus, organize, motivate, manage emotions, and remember details; this is a crucial aspect of each person's journey toward unraveling ADHD.

Individuals with ADHD have a higher heightened sensitivity to environmental stimuli and a more difficult time separating the various information presented to their brains.

As we established in Myth #1, there is no definitive medical test for ADHD, and the disorder exists on a spectrum. Therefore, self-reported traits are all that doctors have to go on when making a diagnosis.

What's important is accepting that the way you see the world is a genuine reflection of how your brain is wired. It is helpful to understand strategies for managing the symptoms of ADHD whether or not you have been formally diagnosed with the disorder.

ADHD Myth #3: ADHD isn't serious.

In most cases, people with ADHD will tell you that their condition has significantly impacted their lives, both positively and negatively.

Problems with learning, family life, school, employment, social relationships, and even driving safety can arise from untreated ADHD. In addition, there is a high correlation between having ADHD and experiencing various psychological and learning difficulties, including anxiety, sadness, and addiction.

Individuals who have ADHD may have a significant positive impact on society due to their boundless vitality, inventiveness, and other strengths. Unfortunately, many famous people struggle with ADHD. People with ADHD tend to be drawn to high-stress careers like the creative arts, sports, business, medicine, and politics.

Celebrities such as Jim Carrey, Ryan Gosling, Woody Harrelson, Michelle Rodriguez, and Will Smith, as well as Justin Timberlake, Sir Richard Branson, Pulitzer Prize-winning journalist Katherine Ellison, celebrity chef Jamie Oliver, political consultant James Carville, Olympic gold-medal winner Michael Phelps, JetBlue founder David Neeleman, Kinko's founder Paul Orfalea, baseball player Pete Rose, and inventor Dean Kamen, are all living with ADHD.

ADHD Myth #4: People with ADHD can't concentrate on anything.

The term ADHD is incredibly deceptive. Persons with ADHD do not suffer from a "deficit" of attention. On the contrary, you pay close attention and could even be hyper-attuned to the subtlest environmental cues.

Concentration is key. In journalist Jonah Lehrer's words, having ADHD means you have less command over your "mental spotlight."

If you're really into something, you might be able to "hyperfocus" on it to the exclusion of all else and give it your undivided attention. This concentration level is common while pursuing anything that truly interests you, whether a passion project, a challenging problem, a field of study, a creative activity, a video game, etc.

However, most of the time, your Focus is likely shaky and readily diverted by other distractions. As a result, you can feel like your thoughts never cease, constantly forget what others are telling you, and you constantly start new projects that you never get around to finishing.

This difference is neurobiological. Dopamine is released in response to engaging in something particularly intriguing or rewarding, which helps make up for the dopamine deficiency in ADHD, resulting in enhanced Focus and drive.

Similarly, your brain may release more dopamine when you're under pressure to complete a task fast because of a looming deadline or because you fear something unpleasant would happen otherwise.

We're exaggerating a bit, but this is the fundamental cause of selective attention in persons with ADHD. In some conditions, particular to each person, they can use their executive functions quite effectively, but they struggle in most other circumstances. They can still achieve great success, though, especially if they focus on what they do best and learn to surround themselves with positive influences.

ADHD Myth #5: Those suffering from it must exert more effort.

Like bad eyesight or an erectile problem, executive functioning in your brain is not something you have complete control over. You can't force yourself to overcome the limitations of ADHD in executive function; this myth is debunked in Myth #4.

If you have symptoms of ADHD, you've undoubtedly heard this message many times, either from others or from your inner monologue:

- It would help if you worked on your willpower, that's all.
- If your mind is set on it, you can focus.
- You're lazy.
- You don't give a damn about this stuff.
- Quit procrastinating and get the job done already!

Because of their experience, people with ADHD know that they can concentrate and perform better in some settings than others, making it simple to trust these claims. You may be hard on yourself for various offenses, such as forgetfulness, tardiness, emotional swings, etc.

In reality, ADHD cannot be cured by sheer force of will. People often feel more defeated and stressed when trying to overcome obstacles by exerting extra effort. Concentrating on the positive and expanding on the events that already hold one's interest can be more beneficial than ignoring one's ADHD symptoms.

ADHD Myth #6: Intelligent people don't need professional help.

Individuals of different IQs can be affected by ADHD, but those with higher IQs are more likely to go undiagnosed. They usually manage to keep their symptoms under wraps. They get by academically despite distraction, procrastination, or lack of Focus.

The key to a fulfilling professional life is finding one's true calling. However, things go downhill if their ADHD is never diagnosed. Like everyone else, they need assistance and support.

Dr. Thomas Brown, the author of Smart But Stuck, has "one of my main interests over the years" in very intelligent young people and adults. But unfortunately, they taught me that intelligence is no defense against attention problems.

It's not only feasible for people with a high IQ to have ADHD, but they're also more likely to go untreated for a longer period since their loved ones believe (incorrectly) that no one with such a high IQ could have the disorder.

In his book, Brown examines the lives of those with ADHD who ranked in the top 9 percent on IQ testing but were otherwise unable to move on. Patients sought help because they were stuck in "chronically unproductive, self-defeating patterns of emotions, cognition, and action," he writes.

They felt confined in their day-to-day interactions with school, work, friends, and family. Their experiences highlight the ongoing challenges people with ADHD have when attempting to maintain self-control and emotional balance.

The following remark from a member of an Unpacking ADHD group conveys the anguish of living with undiagnosed ADHD and the hope of addressing its effects.

I've managed to have a great career while keeping my ADHD symptoms a secret. Nonetheless, the price tag has been extremely high. After learning I have ADHD, I also learned how isolated I am and how little confidence I have in myself.

My understanding and acceptance of my ADHD symptoms have greatly increased thanks to the encouragement of my fellow Unpacking ADHD journey participants. Putting forth my authentic self in the world is something I'm working on. It's Patti Q.

ADHD Myth #7: Medication can cure ADHD.

While ADHD medication is not a cure, it can be helpful. Medication provided for persons with ADHD can greatly aid in managing troublesome features for roughly 80% of those diagnosed.

Several doctors liken taking ADHD meds to wearing glasses to correct eyesight impairments. But, unfortunately, the impact won't last forever. Like wearing your glasses, you need to take your medication for it to have an effect continuously.

Medications for ADHD, in contrast to glasses, rarely provide a "20/20" answer. Successful management of ADHD can need a combination of medication, education, support, counseling, and lifestyle adjustments.

Medications for attention deficit hyperactivity disorder (ADHD) are complex and always changing. Unfortunately, many doctors lack the necessary expertise to guide you in selecting the optimal medication combination for ADHD. For instance, your doctor may recommend an antidepressant instead of a stimulant, despite the latter's potential for better results.

Dr. Charles Parker, the author of New ADHD Medication Rules, asserts that it is incredibly difficult to translate the theory behind ADHD medication into practical, step-by-step instructions for use in the workplace. "Even the most enlightened observer is aware that no rule book specifies what treatments are allowed, what they should accomplish, and how their success should be evaluated."

A little context can be gained from Unpacking ADHD creator Don Baker's personal experience:

When I first tried taking the drug, it had no effect. For the past ten years, I've had to control my ADHD symptoms by strictly monitoring my nutrition, sleep schedule, and other forms of self-care. On the other hand, the medicine worked well when I finally gave it another shot. It doesn't help my ADHD, but it has me doing things I'd rather not.

What you go through won't be the same. However, suppose you do decide to attempt medication for your ADHD. In that case, engaging with a clinical physician familiar with the disorder and the most current treatment options is important.

ADHD Myth #8: It Never Affects Adults.

The percentage of individuals diagnosed with attention deficit hyperactivity disorder has risen over the previous two decades. ADHD is a real condition that can affect people of any age, even adults. Adult-onset ADHD does not exist, though. Unfortunately, many people who exhibit ADHD symptoms as children retain those characteristics as adults.

It has been estimated that between 40 and 70% of children with ADHD keep showing ADHD features in adulthood, and in 2011, the CDC reported that 11 percent of children ages 4 to 17 (6.4 million) had been diagnosed with ADHD.

It is unknown how many youngsters go without a diagnosis or how many people have lived with untreated ADHD their whole lives. According to a 2006 Harvard research financed by the NIMH, 4.4% of U.S. adults between 18 and 44 had signs of ADHD. A much higher real prevalence is possible.

After having a child diagnosed with ADHD or seeking treatment for a related issue like anxiety or depression, many adults realize they also have ADHD.

ADHD Myth #9: Adults with ADHD suffer from constant stimulation due to too much information.

One common misconception about today's youth is that they all have Attention Deficit Hyperactivity Disorder (ADHD) due to the pressures of modern living. But, of course, Facebook is to blame for this mess. With so many distractions around us, it's hard to concentrate.

The information age may be stressful for most people's minds, but it cannot trigger attention deficit hyperactivity disorder (ADHD).

While it's true that everyone may relate to at least one symptom of ADHD, those who live with the condition face daily struggles that go well beyond basic overstimulation. People living with ADHD "pay a significantly larger price for their distracted periods, and it occurs much more often," according to psychologist and author Ari Tuckman, PsyD.

ADHD, which isn't fake, is caused by different neurobiological factors. Individuals with ADHD have an impaired ability to prioritize and organize information due to underactive functioning in the brain's management system. As a result, the intensity of their sensory responses and the efficiency with which they analyze them is increased. Environmental factors cannot be held solely responsible for the development of ADHD, while they may enhance or worsen the disorder.

Myth #10: Everyone with ADHD is hyperactive (and most of them are male).

Hyperactivity is often the most noticeable symptom of attention deficit hyperactivity disorder. Boys are typically portrayed as hyperactive and "bouncing off the walls." Hyperactivity, however, is not a hallmark of all people with ADHD. Some people have problems paying attention, staying on task, and controlling their impulses.

In this respect, gender is an important factor. Females with ADHD tend to be less hyperactive and experience greater depression and anxiety due to the disorder. As a result, women have ADHD at the same rate as men but are much less likely to receive a diagnosis.
This perpetuates the false belief that only boys can have attention deficit hyperactivity disorder (ADHD), as females are more prone to exhibit inattentive rather than hyperactive symptoms.
According to Dr. Kathleen Nadeau, depression is the leading pre-ADD diagnosis for women. The number of times I've had ladies come into my office stating, "I've been in therapy for years, and I've been diagnosed with anxiety and depression, but I'm still having problems" is beyond my capacity to count. It's frustrating because it's a treatable mental illness. That can't be explained away in any way.
Fewer women get diagnosed with ADHD, and many who go undiagnosed often suffer in silence into adulthood. To paraphrase what Nadeau says: "The pressure on women to be organized, self-controlled, to be the one who's keeping everybody else organized is a societal expectation that is deeply established.

CHAPTER 7. HABITS THAT CAN HELP YOU MANAGE ADHD

The 11 million people in the United States with adult attention deficit hyperactivity disorder know how challenging it can be to focus on a single task simultaneously. However, you can learn to manage your ADHD and achieve more success and happiness with the help of treatment and changes to your behavior.

These easy-to-implement techniques can help you control your symptoms so that you can concentrate and flourish.

Symptoms of attention deficit hyperactivity disorder (ADHD), such as distractibility, impulsivity, disorganization, restlessness, overactivity, lack of Focus, and trouble with behavioral control, often begin before age 12 and worsen over time.

You are not alone if you are over 18 and have these symptoms. For many people, attention deficit hyperactivity disorder (ADHD) doesn't end when they reach adulthood. The NIMH estimates that little over 8 percent of American adults (ages 18-44) have been diagnosed with ADHD at some point.

Adults with ADHD often have memory issues, restlessness, and a general inability to focus, in contrast to the impulsivity and hyperactivity that characterize the disorder in children.

Evidence-based therapies such as medication and psychotherapy can be very helpful in managing ADHD, but understanding effective behavioral methods can allow you to regulate your symptoms in the here and now. Here are five methods you may implement immediately to start seeing results.

1. Become Organized

You probably need a new method of an organization if you spend much of the day trying to find out how to get started yet finish up with very little accomplished. By reducing the number of potential sources of stress and making it easier to keep track of your day's activities, an organization can greatly improve your quality of life.

A written schedule for the next day will help you live a more orderly life. Having a plan in place so that you can take charge of your day from the get-go is empowering. In addition, crossing out items on a to-do list that you've already finished is a great way to enhance your mood.

Writing down what needs to be accomplished in the morning might help you get more done throughout the day, whether at work, out and about, or just cleaning the house.

Make it a routine to check your schedule first thing in the morning, again around lunchtime, and one more before bed to see if there are any outstanding items you need to deal with.

The odds of doing everything will increase if similar tasks are grouped. For instance, rather than responding to messages and calls throughout the day, try handling them all in the morning and again in the afternoon. Don't forget to leave some space in your schedule for unforeseen problems.

Tips For Adults With ADHD Who Want To Get Their Houses In Order

Most people, especially those with ADHD, find the prospect of cleaning up their homes and getting organized to be quite daunting. However, adults with ADHD who are organizers benefit from a focused strategy due to their heightened susceptibility to distraction, difficulty making decisions, and challenges with organizing their materials.

- Focus on one room at a time rather than trying to clean the whole house.

- Put aside time in your schedule for cleaning and organizing, but give yourself only thirty minutes to an hour to complete each chore.

- Make piles of things to throw away, things to donate, and things to keep.

- Make sure you schedule some time to drop off your filled donation box. Organize a time and place to drop off the donated things.

- Do not give up on your ambitions without first seeking the assistance of a friendly professional organizer.

Managing Disorganization When You Have ADHD

If you're struggling to keep your ADHD under control, the following suggestions can help you turn to organize into a habit.

- **Use a planner**: For instance, a calendar, planner notebook, or smart device to keep track of your daily obligations.

- **Plan your organization** by adding tasks to your calendar as actionable appointments. Plan on spending 15 minutes at 7 o'clock to straighten up the living room, for instance. Routinely daily. As part of a continuous effort to reduce clutter, set aside half an hour to straighten up your workspace.

- **Make a "home" for items**: Make that spot its permanent residence when you find where something should be. For instance, keep your keys, sunglasses, and wallet in one convenient location by the door and always put them back there.

- **Use labels or color-coding**: This helps to organize your stuff, whether they're for work or home. This helps you find what you need quickly and easily.

2. Maintain A Routine

After getting used to planning your day, settle into a pattern that will help you succeed no matter what comes your way. For example, accustom yourself to placing your keys in the tray as soon as you enter the house. Before entering the living room, please remove your outerwear and place it in the closet. Examine your habits to find the ones that serve you best.

Create habits by establishing procedures to accomplish typical tasks more efficiently. For example, make a list of your weekly necessities and take a few minutes before you leave to add anything else you might need for the upcoming week to the list. This will help you feel less disorganized and more productive while grocery shopping.

How To Create a Routine While Dealing With ADHD

Developing a habit of doing the same thing repeatedly calls for effort and time. Following these guidelines, it will be easier to maintain a routine.

- **Adhere to a mail routine**: Set aside weekly time to open, organize, and keep mail. In addition, set aside a place or container specifically for incoming mail, such as bills, cheques, and insurance documents.

- **Create a chore routine**: Schedule weekly duties such as laundry and dishes on specific days and times.
- **Take advantage of electronic notifications and reminder**s by utilizing your mobile devices, apps, and other smart technologies. Setting alarms and other reminders for scheduled events should become second nature. For example, create notifications to remind you to take your medication or put out the trash.

- **Start an exercise routine**: This can help boost the dopamine levels in your brain, which are often lower than average in people with ADHD. In addition, a person's "executive function," or their ability to plan, organize, and retain information, is enhanced by regular exercise.

3. Make Difficult Tasks Easier To Handle

If you're working on a large, complex project requiring multiple steps and scrutiny, splitting the task into smaller, more achievable steps may be good.

Make sure you don't miss any steps by making a thorough checklist or listing all the various parts of your assignment—no need to prioritize or even write down these tasks at the outset. Then, when you've gotten going, add items and sort them by date or alphabet to keep the momentum going.

ADHD Adults' Guide To Time Management

Though organization and routine lay the groundwork for more efficient time management, diving into a scheduled project can be intimidating. If the scale of your responsibility seems too great, or if you aren't sure where to start, don't worry. Instead, consider using the timer approach to work for brief periods whenever you encounter these emotional or physical obstacles.

Split up big projects into smaller steps. For example, rather than tackling the intimidating chore of "cleaning the entire living room," break it down into manageable chunks by assigning specific tasks such as:

- Load the dishwasher by bringing dishes from the living room.

- Toys should be returned to their bedrooms, and shoes should be put away so that the living room can be used as intended.

- Cleaning the carpet with a vacuum is a must.

- Tables and other surfaces should be wiped off with polish or cleaning spray.

If you need to get a big project rolling, try this out:

- For the next 10 to 15 minutes, focus on only one of the specified activities.

- In those brief moments, you should concentrate on that one task.

- When the alarm goes off, you can continue with the same work for another 10 to 15 minutes or switch to a new one.

- Keep working in 15-minute increments for as long as you can if you're still enthusiastic after that.

- Stop what you're doing if you need to rest, and pick it back up later or the next day.

4. Reduce Distractions

Reducing the number of potential distractions can help you concentrate for long periods on tasks that are important to you professionally or personally. In addition, home environments can be simplified and decluttered to enhance concentration.

At work, simplification is also a boon. Complete ongoing work before taking on new tasks to help you focus.

Tips For Working Professionals With Attention Deficit Hyperactivity Disorder

Where do you find the most office distractions? Those pesky social networks? Have you set up any news alerts? Email? Texts? Your cluttered work area? Coworkers, who like to make a lot of noise?

Working with distractions is a common problem for people with attention deficit hyperactivity disorder (ADHD). First, identify the root causes of your key distractions and work to eliminate them.

- **Turn off notifications**: Calls will be sent to voicemail— Disable alerts for incoming messages if possible. Instead, perform regular, scheduled checks of your messages.
- **Wear noise-canceling headphones**: Try some headphones if you need peace in a noisy setting.

- **Pick somewhere serene**: For instance, a cubicle or office with little noise.

- **Put on some music**: Put on some music or use a white noise machine. There is evidence that the linearity and rhythmic understanding of the ADHD brain can be improved by listening to structured music. Yet, not every music operates in the same fashion.

Some adults with ADHD find lyrically-rich, loud music a major distraction. Classical music and relaxing instrumentals are the greatest choices for improving focus.

- **Change your work schedule**: Begin earlier or later than normal when the office is calmer.

- **Keep your workspace neat**: Don't let a mess distract you from your work.

5. Recognize Your Limits

It's normal to wake up with high hopes for the productive and enjoyable time you'll have today. However, taking on more responsibilities than they can handle or failing to allow enough time to complete chores causes stress for several people.

Putting extra effort above your capabilities consistently is a surefire way to stress oneself out. When you don't follow through on commitments you make, whether to yourself, your employer, your loved ones, or anybody else, it can deflate your spirits and leave you feeling more disorganized than you already were.

One important part of managing ADHD is recognizing when you've hit your limit and need to start saying "no" to things. When you know and accept your limitations, you can make better decisions and follow through on fewer commitments.

6. Eat Right

The risk of becoming overweight is increased in those with ADHD. Unfortunately, professionals have a hard time putting their finger on a reason. Considering that your food may not be a high priority for you. Worse, you might not realize when you're full. Snacking and overeating are two common results of either of these.

Confer with your physician if you need help figuring out how to start eating better. They'll link you up with an ADHD-specialized nutritionist.

To help you get started, consider the following:

- **Eat a wide range of nutritious foods every day.** However, no one meal or nutrient can help your condition. It would help if you instead ate the same minimally processed diet recommended for adults.

Put these on your plate.

- Veggies and fruit.
- Whole grains.
- Healthy unsaturated fats.
- Lean protein.
- **Do some planning**. There's a risk that you'll neglect your diet if you're preoccupied. Then, you could make hasty, unhealthy decisions when mealtime rolls along. Plan your meals in advance and always have healthy options available to make life easy.

More tips for your weekly menu:

- Get a list together and head off to the supermarket.
- Prepare enough food for leftovers.
- Make things like soup that can be frozen for later.
- Prepare fresh veggies for chopping in advance.
- Go out and purchase some frozen veggies and fruit.
- Maintain a supply of staples like brown rice and beans.

- **Avoid eating trigger foods**. Hyperactivity disorder is not caused by what you eat. However, your symptoms could be influenced by certain ingredients. For example, some people have issues using artificial flavors, colors, and other additives.

This, however, is not supported by substantial evidence. So instead, keep a diary to track how you feel before, during, and after eating. Consult a nutritionist if you're unsure what to do.

7. Exercise

There is mounting proof that exercise can help reduce the effects of attention deficit hyperactivity disorder. The release of endorphins, dopamine, and norepinephrine during exercise is a major theory for this phenomenon. Stimulant medicines, the standard treatment for attention deficit hyperactivity disorder, work by altering the levels of these substances in the brain.

People with ADHD, like all adults, benefit from exercising at least 30 minutes, 5 days per week. Jogging and fast walking are examples of moderate activity. Although it raises the heart rate, it shouldn't interfere with the normal conversational flow.

Adults with attention deficit hyperactivity disorder (ADHD) may gain by engaging in physical activity in the ways listed below.

- Relieve some pressure.
- Improve people's health and happiness.
- The ability to regulate one's impulses needs improvement.
- Get rid of your hyperactivity.
- Improve your capacity for organizing and completing tasks.

8. Get Sufficient Sleep

The average adult needs between 7 and 9 hours of sleep per night. Those with attention deficit hyperactivity disorder may struggle with falling asleep or staying asleep (ADHD). Sleep disturbances may exacerbate your existing symptoms.

If you are having trouble sleeping, talk to your doctor. It may be essential to adjust the time of day you take your medicine or try a new medication altogether. Of course, any underlying problems will also be investigated.

It's possible that getting treatment for one of the following health issues can help you sleep better:

- Insomnia.
- Stress or depression.
- Issues with the circadian rhythm (your sleep-wake cycle).
- Obstructive sleep apnea.
- Restless legs syndrome.
- Narcolepsy.

You can improve your sleep by adopting these practices:

- Keep away from alcohol and caffeine.
- Try to work out, but don't do it just before bed.
- Maintain a regular sleep-wake schedule.
- Try to avoid taking naps in the late afternoon.
- A weighted blanket can help.

You may want to contact a sleep doctor if that doesn't work. Biofeedback, relaxation training, and cognitive behavioral therapy for insomnia are a few other options.

9. Stop Engaging In Unhealthy Behavior

To alleviate your problems, you may resort to harmful behaviors. If you have ADHD, however, it may be helpful to skip or reduce participation in some events. The following are included in that category:

Drug and alcohol use. Just don't do drugs. To deal with the challenges of ADHD in adulthood, some people turn to substances like marijuana and alcohol. However, some people taking ADHD drugs may compare the effects of nicotine and cocaine and report feeling the same benefits. However, those who have ADHD are more likely to develop a dependency on these drugs.

Smoking cigarettes. You may increase your child's risk of developing attention deficit hyperactivity disorder (ADHD) if you smoke during pregnancy. In addition, folks with ADHD are twice as likely to be smokers as those without it. It could be quite difficult to stop once you get started.

See a doctor if you need assistance stopping. Medication for ADHD is one form of treatment. Don't give up if your first attempt fails. Among stimulants, nicotine is among the most habit-forming. Most people need more than one try to kick the habit finally.

A lot of digital screen time. A smartphone is something you probably can't live without. Though you shouldn't abuse it, moderation in use is advised. Some research suggests that those with ADHD are at a higher risk of becoming "smartphone addicted."

Some studies suggest that more teenage screen use increases the risk of developing ADHD in later life. However, it is unclear whether or not this behavior is linked to ADHD symptoms in professional assessments.

10. Handle Stress

Problems with attention and focus during a normal day are expected for those with ADHD. However, stress may exacerbate the symptoms as well. Having that added pressure can make it much more difficult to concentrate or keep your emotions in check.

Discuss with your healthcare provider about including stress management in your therapy. Some possible advice and approaches they may offer are as follows:

- Make a plan and break down the job into manageable chunks.
- Make use of a calendar to plot out your schedule.
- Stick to routines.
- The practice of mindfulness meditation is recommended.
- Practice deep breathing and other relaxation techniques to calm down.
- Attempt cognitive behavioral therapy.

If you need assistance, don't be reluctant to ask for it. You are not alone; many individuals have been where you are. Talk to your doctor or social worker for recommendations for a group like this.

11. Consider Your Wins

When asked about regrets, Beth Main, a certified ADHD coach and founder of ADHD Solutions. advised, "Don't spend all your time thinking about what you didn't accomplish or couldn't do before." The alternative, she advised, was to reflect on the day's successes and achievements before turning it in.

Something as easy as "organized my day," "exercised," or "made the first step on a project I have been putting off" can count.

12. Talk To Yourself Positively

Mind your self-talk. Negative remarks should be disputed, and positive ones should be used in their stead.

As we believe our own words, they come to fruition.

Say, for example, your boss assigns you a new task in the office. You naturally tell yourself negative things like "I'll never get this done" or "I'm a failure." Instead, you should say something like, "I'm capable, and I can do this project on time."

13. Use Money Management Software

Money management problems are a major issue for adults with ADHD, according to Sarkis. She gave a few examples, including people who have trouble keeping track of important financial documents, who don't save money, and who make impulsive purchases.

Having a software tool to manage your accounts is a tremendous assistance when trying to keep everything straight. Quicken and Mint are two software examples Sarkis recommended since they "update themselves with your financial information and can store your information in the 'cloud' so it is never lost."

(She recommended consulting with a financial advisor as well. Consult an expert in your problem area (such as financial planning, tax preparation, controlling your spending habits, or saving for retirement).

14. Get Yourself A Accountability Pal

Adults with ADHD may also struggle with a lack of structure and accountability. Wright, co-author of Fidget to Focus, gave the example of college students transitioning from having very scheduled days in high school to essentially no structure in college.

Hire an ADHD coach, form an accountability group with friends, or work with a group of people to hold each other accountable, she advised.

Take the case of the woman who struggled to do her daily housework. Per their arrangement, she'd do chores for her pal on Saturday mornings before they went out to lunch. Unfortunately, she wasn't prepared the first time, so her companion left. After that, she never missed another Saturday."

15. Always Look On The Bright Side; Today Is A Brand New Day

Anyone can attest that establishing a new routine is difficult and fraught with setbacks. Main argued that it is impossible for anyone, with or without ADHD, to create a habit in a single day and maintain it flawlessly indefinitely.

She warned that there may be times when I would "forget," "get sidetracked," or "simply not care." However, you should always keep in mind that "today is a brand fresh day." You can begin over by pressing the "reset" button.

Consider what you can take away from it and how you may improve for tomorrow. Then proceed.

Eventually, with consistent practice, these routines will become automatic, as Sarkis put it. Stop being so hard on yourself. You've been dealing with ADHD all your life; things could take time to improve.

CHAPTER 8. HOW TO OVERCOME ADULT ADHD

Although we discussed habits that can help you manage ADHD as an adult, this chapter is an extension of it. You'll be learning how to overcome it. The effects of ADD/ADHD are far-reaching and can affect every aspect of a person's existence. These strategies, however, will aid in alleviating symptoms, enhancing concentration, and restoring order where there was once just chaos.

Dealing With Adult ADHD (Or ADD)

Making payments on time, keeping up with job and family obligations, and maintaining social relationships can all feel impossible for someone with attention deficit hyperactivity disorder (ADHD), formerly known as ADD.

Adults with ADHD face unique difficulties which can harm their health, personal relationships, and careers. Due to your symptoms, you may have significant procrastination, difficulty keeping to deadlines, and impulsive actions. It's possible, too, that you feel like your loved ones just don't get it.

You can take charge of your ADHD symptoms by learning new skills. The habits you form daily are the foundation upon which your success is built.

By identifying and capitalizing on your strengths, you may enhance your productivity, efficiency, and social interactions at work. In addition, as you work to improve yourself, you may share your story with others so they may better empathize with your situation.

Yet, transformation is not an overnight process. A positive view, perseverance, and practice are essential components of self-help for ADHD. However, these methods can help you accomplish more, feel more in charge of your life, and boost your confidence.

Guidelines For Organizing And Managing Clutter

Adults with ADHD often struggle with staying organized due to the disorder's hallmark symptoms of impulsivity and fidgetiness. If you have ADHD, becoming organized at work or home could make you feel like you're drowning.

With experience, you might learn to break down daunting tasks into more manageable parts and arrange your resources systematically. You may set yourself up to maintain organization and control clutter by establishing various structures and routines and using resources like daily planners and reminders.

1. Create and maintain order and cleanliness.

Start by sorting everything in your room, house, or office into categories, then decide what you absolutely need and what can be put away or thrown away. Next, form a routine of making notes and lists to help you stay organized and keep your freshly established order with consistent everyday habits.

- **Create space**. Think about what you use most frequently, and put the rest in boxes or a closet. Please ensure you put keys, bills, and often misplaced objects in their designated spots. Get rid of clutter by throwing away unnecessary items.

- **Make use of a day planner or calendar app**. You can keep track of your appointments and other events with the help of a day planner or a digital calendar on your phone or computer. If you use an electronic calendar, you can create reminders that will pop up on your device to help you remember important dates.

- **Use lists**. Use lists and reminders to stay on top of your appointments, projects, deadlines, and other commitments. If you're going to utilize a planner, that's where you should place your to-do lists and other notes. You have a wealth of options on your computer or mobile device. Start looking for task managers and apps with "to-do" lists.

- **Get over it already**. Doing things like filing files, cleaning up messes, or answering phone calls right away, rather than putting them off until later, will help you remember what you plan to do and keep you from being distracted. If anything can be done in less than two minutes, you shouldn't put it off.

2. Control your paper trail.

Some people with ADHD are particularly disorganized when it comes to paper tasks. Finally, however, you may end the never-ending stacks of mail and papers that seem to accumulate on your kitchen counter, desk, or office floor. Setting up a paper system that serves your needs is simple.

- **Take care of mail regularly**. Once you bring the mail inside daily, set aside a few minutes to sort through it. A specific location for mail allows you to quickly and easily discard unwanted items, file important documents, or take necessary action.

- **Give up the paper and go digital**. Reduce the piles of paper you have to sort through. Make the switch to paperless billing by requesting electronic statements and receipts. In the United States, the Direct Marketing Association (DMA) offers a Mail Preference Service to help eliminate unwanted mail.

- **Make a filing system**. Different sorts of paperwork with dividers or file folders (such as medical records, receipts, and income statements). Suppose you want to find something in your files fasts, label and color-code them.

Advice on How to Manage Your Time and Keep to Your Schedule

ADHD frequently causes problems with organizing one's time effectively. As a result, you may have trouble keeping track of time, routinely miss important deadlines, avoid strenuous activities, delay, or perform tasks out of sequence.

Adults with ADHD often "hyperfocus" on a single activity to the exclusion of all others, leading to a frustrating lack of productivity. As a result, you may feel helpless and incompetent, and others may become irritated due to these challenges. But there are ways to improve your time management.

1. Tips on managing your time.

It's common for adults with ADD to have a skewed perception of time. One of the oldest methods for synchronizing one's internal clock with the rest of the world is simply buying a clock.

- **Learn to keep track of time**. You should maintain track of the time using a wristwatch or a large, easily readable clock. Make sure you record the time you begin working on a task, either verbally or in writing.
- **Set timers**. You should set a timer or alarm to remind you when your allotted time for a task has expired. Setting the alarm off at predetermined intervals might help you stay focused and aware of how much time has passed throughout longer jobs.

- **It's always better to give oneself extra time than less**. Unfortunately, adults with attention deficit hyperactivity disorder (ADHD) are notoriously lousy at timing themselves. So give yourself an extra ten minutes for every thirty you anticipate needing to get somewhere or finish a task.

- **Set reminders and plan to arrive early**. For example, put the start time of your appointments fifteen minutes sooner than they are. To avoid rushing around trying to find your keys or phone when it's time to leave, set alarms to get you out the door on time.

2. Suggestions for setting priorities.

Adults with ADHD have trouble maintaining focus and frequently switch gears, making it challenging to get things done and especially daunting to tackle huge assignments. Therefore, to go around this:

- **You must prioritize your tasks**. Consider what needs to be done first and foremost, and work your way down.

- **Just take it slow and easy**. Make complex tasks more manageable by breaking them down into smaller ones.
- **Focus on what you're doing**. To keep from going off track, setting a timer for specific periods can be helpful.

3. Develop the ability to say no.

Adults with ADHD may say "yes" to too many professional or social commitments because of their impulsive nature. However, having too much on your plate might cause you to feel stressed out and exhausted, which will show in your job.

The ability to get things done, uphold social commitments, and maintain a healthy lifestyle may all benefit from learning to say no. However, before saying yes to something new, be sure you have enough time for it.

Advice On Managing Your Money And Bills

Many persons with ADHD find it difficult to handle their finances since it necessitates budgeting, planning, and organization. In addition, adults with ADHD may have trouble using conventional financial management methods because they demand too much effort, paperwork, and precision.

By developing a straightforward and reliable system, you may control your money and end wasteful spending, late fees, and other consequences of procrastination.

1. Control your budget.

Step one in gaining control of your budget is to take an honest look at your current financial status. Then, get started with budgeting by keeping track of your spending for a month. It will be much easier to track your spending this way.

Keeping track of all the money you waste on frivolous purchases might be eye-opening. This snapshot of your spending patterns can inform a monthly budget calculated from your income and other relevant factors.

Learn to control your spending to stay within your set limits. For example, suppose you spend too much money on eating out. In that case, one option is to establish a plan for eating, considering the necessary resources and time for grocery shopping and cooking.

2. Create a basic strategy for managing your finances and paying your bills.

Create a simple, well-organized system to store paperwork and keep track of bills and other financial obligations. The convenience of online banking can be a godsend for those with attention deficit hyperactivity disorder. When finances are organized digitally, there is less need for paperwork, less chance of mistakes, and fewer lost slips.

- **It would help if you started doing your banking online**. With online banking, you can eliminate the guesswork from budgeting. In addition, your online account balance will be updated every day after being checked against the previous day's closing balance.

In addition to setting up recurring monthly payments, you can also pay irregular or one-off expenses whenever you like. The best thing is that there is no risk of lost mail or overdue fines.

- **Create reminders for paying bills**. Even if you'd rather not set up automatic payments, electronic reminders can help you stay on top. You can, for example, use your calendar app or set

- **Utilize modern technology**. Take advantage of the many free programs to better manage your money. Creating one may take some time, but once it's connected to your other accounts, they'll be kept up to date without any further input from you. These tools can simplify your finance management.

3. Stop impulsive buying.

Shopping and impulsivity caused by ADHD can be highly risky. It has the potential to cause financial hardship as well as emotional distress. However, with some planning, you can avoid making impulsive purchases.

- Don't bring your checkbook or credit card; use cash.

- Get rid of all your credit cards but one. Instead, prepare a shopping list of necessities and stick to it.

- Keep track of your spending with a calculator (pro tip: your phone has one) while you shop.

- Avoid stores where you're inclined to overspend, discard catalogs as they come, and stop receiving emails from retailers.

How To Maintain Concentration And Get More Done At Work

When it comes to the workplace, people with ADHD face unique difficulties. Every day, you're probably expected to perform the most difficult things: stay organized, finish work, sit still, and listen calmly.

While it may be difficult to manage ADHD and a demanding profession, you can make the most of your strengths while reducing the impact of your symptoms by making adjustments to your working environment.

1. Organize your workplace.

Take baby steps toward a more orderly workplace, cubicle, or desk. Then, adopt the following practices to maintain order:

- **Schedule some time every day to keep things in order**. It's important to clear your desk and put things in order daily; spending more than five or ten minutes doing so can help you focus. Try keeping items out of sight by placing them in drawers or bins on your desk.

- **Use colors and lists**. People with ADHD can benefit greatly from color coding. Write things down if you tend to forget.

- **Prioritize**. Prioritizing your projects by importance can help you get things done faster and more efficiently. Even if they are only for yourself, timelines should be set for everything.

2. Remove distractions

The place of work and surrounding environment can substantially impact productivity for those with attention difficulties. Share with your coworkers that you need to focus, and use these strategies to block off distractions:

- **Your workplace has an impact**. Without an office of your own, you might be able to accomplish your task in a vacant meeting room or other workplace. If you're in a lecture hall or conference, try to get a seat near the presenter and far from those who talk throughout the presentation.

- **Reduce external noise**. Place your desk against a wall and try to avoid unnecessary clutter. Posting a "Do Not Disturb" sign is always available to deter unwanted visitors.

Do things like let voicemail take calls and get back to callers when they leave messages, disable your email and social media accounts during specific times of the day, or even go offline entirely. Noise-canceling headphones or a white-noise generator are good options if ambient noise is a problem.

- **Put off the big ideas for now**. Do you know how you can't seem to stop yourself from being sidetracked by brilliant ideas or strange ideas? Don't forget to jot down these ideas (or save them to your phone) for subsequent consideration. Some persons with ADHD find that reviewing their notes at the end of the day helps them relax and wind down.

3. Increase your attention span.

It's not that you can't focus as an adult with ADHD; it's simply that you could have a hard time doing so, especially if the task at hand isn't particularly interesting.

Adults with ADHD may have difficulty sitting through tedious meetings or lectures. Likewise, persons with ADHD may struggle to juggle many directives. So here are some ways to sharpen your attention and response time:

- **Could you write it down?** Request a copy of the necessary documents, such as a meeting agenda or lecture outline, in advance of any meeting, lecture, workshop, or other events that require your undivided attention.

Take notes and pay attention during the meeting by consulting your prepared documents. Taking notes while listening will help you pay closer attention to what is being said.

- **Echo directions**. Say back the directions loudly to double-check that you understood them.

- **Move around**. If you find yourself getting antsy or fidgety, getting up and moving around at strategic intervals can help. You can squeeze a stress ball, for instance, during a meeting as long as you don't make too much noise. Likewise, if you're having trouble focusing during a meeting, try getting up and moving about between breaks.

Ways to Reduce Stress and Feel Better

The impulsivity and disorganization that characterize ADHD can make it difficult to maintain a regular sleep routine, eat well, or get enough exercise, all of which add to the burden of the disorder and can make you feel down and out. Taking responsibility for your life and establishing positive new routines is the most effective strategy to break the pattern.

Maintaining serenity, lessening the frequency and severity of mood fluctuations, and reducing the impact of anxiety and depression can all be aided by eating healthily, sleeping enough, and exercising regularly.

Consistent routines can make life more manageable, while adopting healthier behaviors can lessen the severity of ADHD symptoms, including impulsivity, hyperactivity, and inability to focus.

1. Get some fresh air and exercise.

Exercising is one of the best and most effective ways to treat ADHD symptoms like hyperactivity and impulsivity. Working out pent-up stress, negative emotions, and aggressive tendencies via physical activity is a great way to improve mental health, strengthen relationships, and provide stability.

Exercise every day. Pick an activity, such as a team sport or a workout routine you can do with a friend that is both challenging and enjoyable.

ADHD patients frequently feel better in the fresh air and greenery of the outdoors.

Try calming workouts like yoga, tai chi, or mindful strolling. They are effective stress relievers and help you learn to regulate your thoughts and actions.

2. Get enough sleep.

Adults with ADHD may find that their symptoms worsen when they don't get enough sleep, making it more difficult to handle stress and stay on task throughout the day. Adjustments to your daily routine can enhance a restful night's sleep.

- It's best to lay off caffeine in the evening.

- Intense, consistent exercise is recommended, but not within the hour before bed.

- Develop a consistent and relaxing "bedtime" ritual, such as a warm shower or bath before turning in.

- Keep a consistent sleep-wake cycle, even on days off.

3. Eat healthily.

Though poor diet is not the direct cause of ADHD, it can worsen the condition. Changing what and how you eat can dramatically affect your concentration, vitality, and stress levels.

- Consume many modest meals daily.
- Don't eat as much candy and fast food as you can help it.
- Be sure to eat a good amount of protein at each meal.
- Try to get several servings of whole grains into your diet daily, as they are an excellent source of fiber.

4. Practice mindfulness.

Constant practice of mindfulness meditation can do more than help you relax; it can also strengthen your ability to ignore distractions, rein in your impulses, sharpen your focus, and give you command over your feelings. Some adults with ADHD may find meditation difficult due to hyperactive symptoms, but taking it gradually can help.

Try meditating for brief periods at first, then as you become used to it and improve your concentration, work up to longer sessions. The trick is to use these mindfulness strategies regularly to never stray from your path. Finally, try out some guided meditation applications or websites, especially if they are free or cheap.

CHAPTER 9. REAL-LIFE EXAMPLE OF A MAN WITH AN UNDIAGNOSED ADHD

This chapter will show you the life story of men with undiagnosed ADHD and the dangers involved. This is why you should try as much as possible to seek help concerning your ADHD.

Dylan Rosen

If you're searching for an "ADHD Success Story," stop reading now. Neither Michael Phelps' gold medal haul nor Terry Bradshaw's arm's length gives me an unfair advantage. From the day I stepped foot in first grade till now, at 30, my life has been a series of ups and downs. Nevertheless, if you're interested in reading about someone's real and honest account of growing up with undiagnosed ADHD, I invite you to keep reading.

A Quiet Battle

My ADHD symptoms were as iconic as the Rolling Stones to rock music when I was in elementary school. But overall, I think I did very well. My educators consistently remarked on my IQ.

Middle school was another time I excelled academically; I even made the president's list.

A few things shifted as I transitioned from middle school to high school. My report card dropped from an A- to a D-. So did the nature of my friendships and romantic partnerships.

In addition to losing touch with long-time acquaintances, I stopped making new ones. I considered myself an introvert and a hermit. My self-confidence was dwindling, and I could taste the nastiness of despair in the air.

The academic requirements at my school were putting an intolerable amount of stress on me. When added to the constant criticism I faced at home, I struggled to cope with the stress.

Academic success was a must for me to please my parents. My parents threatened to send me to technical school when I brought home a terrible midterm report one semester. Where I grew up, going to a vocational school was viewed as the ultimate admission of defeat.

Isolated And Feeling Like A Failure

Why didn't my parents recognize that I was making an effort? When I tried to do my homework, I'd grow bored and move on to something more interesting, like a video game. Despite my best efforts, reading always puts me to sleep.

My academic life started to become entangled with other things. My inability to control my schedule was a major flaw of mine. As a result, I could not focus or make decisions about the future.

Tasks for the future, such as projects, become dreadful. I couldn't think of a way to make it happen. Yet, such skills are crucial while studying complex topics like DNA or Julius Caesar.

At 15, I felt alone and like a complete failure. When I felt inadequate, I cried a lot. Myd punched me when she wasn't yelling at Finally when, when I turned sixteen, I left her house and started living with my dad. My life improved as a result of this.

But now my grades are better because of it.

It Seemed Like No One Noticed My Attempts

My father had the same attitude toward my academic performance as my mother and stepfather. So, as a result, even if I gave it my all, I could only be what was not good enough.

I n't shake the feeling that I wasn't giving it my all. For some reason, my father was unable to recognize my efforts. When doing chemistry work, I'd stop when I felt the familiar drowsiness in my eyes.

That I was a letdown and a disappointment weighed heavily on my mind, and I felt shame for feeling this way. Likewise, I experienced a recurring sense of isolation throughout my life.

I was damaged by years of criticism and reminders of my shortcomings. The world had already made its statement: You got all A's but still got a C in math.
So, I hobbled into community college.

Similar discussions occurred in college that had begun in high school. I dropped out of school for fewters and got failing grades in several courses. I was hard on myself because I did not finish school like most friends and family.

It took me five years to finish my associate's degree. By this time, I already had a spouse.

Challenges Worsened, But They Were Not Yet Prepared To "Seek Treatment"

The depression I'd been experiencing just worsened, and dealing with it was a constant effort. My new marriage and my performance at work suffered due to my depression. But unfortunately, there was still no way I could get help.

Within the first few months of my marriage, I started having problems at work. Perhaps I was not learning the ropes fast enough, leading to my dismissal from my previous position. In a previous job, I frequently was screamed at for things like being slow to grasp a concept or unable to locate a specific instrument.

The frequently shouting manager was always ready to pounce on me. Of course, I didn't intend to be a bad worker. But, the entire time, I felt terrible about myself, like I was lost in a desert with no other humans around.

To add insult to injury, I started feeling anxious around this time.

The Path from Chaos to Light

My wife and I ended our marriage after around three years. What happened after that altered my whole existence.

My anxiety issues first led me to my family doctor in the summer of 2006. I also visited a therapist who helped me identify my life's greatest obstacle.

In our second session together, she informed me that my answers to a questionnaire confirmed her suspicion that I have ADHD and have done so for my whole life. So finally, like a thirsty traveler who stumbles onto a well in the middle of a desert, my thirst was quenched.

I'm doing fine now, several years later. Now that I've graduated Magna Cum Laude with my Bachelor's degree, I'm the proud owner of an apartment. It was a ten-year process for me. I was laid off the year I completed my degree program. I was falling short in my productivity.

How did I fall through the safety net supposed to protect me?

Recently, I have been wondering why, even before the ADHD diagnosis, they could not communicate with me when I was a child. As a result, I received a barrage of criticism for my academic performance on each report card. Yet, they've always stuck by my side.

I'm living proof of the devastation this condition can cause. I am living proof that no matter how hard you try, it is never enough to make do with what you have. Because of my strained relationship with my mother and inability to live up to her expectations, I always try to make up for my lack of confidence.

Greg

I'm Greg, and I can attest firsthand to the devastation that comes with having undiagnosed ADHD. As a child of the '60s and '70s, I had never heard of ADHD. Reflecting on my chaotic childhood, I realize my parents suffered from ADHD. It's hardly surprising that I inherited ADHD because of how strongly hereditary factors contribute to it.

My parents loved me very much as a kid, although they were frequently preoccupied with other things. As a result, I lacked proper parental supervision and direction and faced many problems.

I was constantly getting in trouble for being a disruptive class participant who constantly interrupted the teacher, never turned in their assignments, and had trouble maintaining attention.

When I misbehaved in class, I either had to sit on a chair outside the classroom during instruction, missed recess, or got paddled (a common practice at the time). My teachers viewed me solely through the lens of a troublemaker.

People labeled me a "bad" kid, so the kids I hung out with naturally shared that label. Then, in middle school, I started smoking pot to calm my mind and help me unwind. Even though it was against the law, I kept smoking weed for the better of my life.

I usually got into problems at school, yet I did well on academic tests. So many of my teachers have told me, "You have so much promise." They didn't think I was being given enough challenges in the classroom. When I acted out in class and didn't do my homework, they put me in a program for "Mentally Gifted Minors," but eventually, I had to leave.

My dad ditched us when I was a senior in high school. Mom had no idea I was dabbling in the dark arts of drug use. I was a junior who struggled in every class and was consequently committed to a juvenile detention center due to my poor performance. I began to change my life for the better by working out with weights while I was in jail.

I got advice on diet and exercise from a school-employed trainer when I had to redo my junior year of high school. I spent numerous hours daily in the school's weight room, where I delighted in the challenging workout. My state of mind was enhanced by physical activity. In my final two years of high school, I was able to think more clearly and achieve perfect grades. Aside from that, I also found decent part-time work.

I didn't pursue further education after high school since I anticipated making this my full-time occupation. Even though I was paid well, I had to work the night shift. That's right; I skipped my last gym session. My ADHD symptoms worsened since I hadn't been getting enough rest or exercising. Anxiety at being naked again filled my body.

Amphetamines alleviated my symptoms such that I could keep working the overnight shift.

The arrest for drug possession and subsequent job loss occurred when I was twenty-four. A felony on my record made it difficult to get a job, so I decided to strike out on my own and open a landscaping business. As a kid, I used to mow lawns, so starting a landscaping business would be a good way to make some quick cash until something better came. Many people liked what I was selling, so I soon expanded.

I married, and we had two kids. The combination of frequent coffee breaks during the day and strenuous physical activity at work helped me maintain my concentration and productivity. To settle my anxious thoughts at night, I started smoking weed. Unfortunately, by the time I was 28, the combined effects of my responsibilities and marijuana had rendered me cognitively incapable of meeting them.

My landscaping company went down because of tax debt and poor management decisions. As a result, my wife, two girls, and I have relocated to my mother's house. She probably wouldn't have refused us, but she probably felt bad about it. As a husband, a parent, and a son, I felt like a total failure.

I enrolled in several self-improvement courses while diligently seeking solutions to my life's problems. As a result, I am now better able to control my moods, have established and stick to regular habits, and limit my diet to healthy options. In addition, I completed my computer science degree because of my improved routines. Even though I put in twice as much work as my classmates, I still graduated near the top of my class.

During my time at the university, I worked as a salesperson. The work environment was conducive to people with attention deficit hyperactivity disorder. All day long, I made sales calls and did very little follow-up or paperwork. In a short time, I was promoted to a higher position and earned more than I would have in a computer science-related field.

I learned a lot about business management from the goods I was selling. Eventually, I launched an enterprise incubator and staffed it with meticulous planners.

Over the years, it expanded to employ over a hundred people and seeded several successful startups. Due to my track record of business success, I was requested to serve as the chairman of CyberTek University, a pioneer in delivering live online instruction.

I bought a beautiful house and had two more daughters at this time of great prosperity. Everyone's predictions about my future potential looked to be coming true. Everything was going fine, but I made multiple errors due to my ADHD. As of 2010, I had no choice but to file for bankruptcy.

After failing miserably on the first attempt, I started over, this time applying what I had learned in the self-improvement classes on controlling my feelings and thoughts. Then, taking the opportunity to further my career, I accepted a position in sales and have since risen through the ranks to become an executive with stock in a promising startup.
But my undiagnosed ADHD made me ill-suited for the role. So a joint decision to have me exit the company in 2019 was reached.

The pandemic created brand new problems. I was unable to visit my regular gym. My normal habits have been disrupted. Repeated episodes of my problematic behavior surfaced. Finally, sometime in 2020, I made an appointment to see a psychiatrist. He correctly diagnosed my ADHD and put me on medication.

My four older daughters were all diagnosed with ADHD not long after I was first diagnosed. I wish I had realized it sooner so we might have avoided so much trouble. I feel terrible that I could not be there for them emotionally as they were growing up; I fear it will leave permanent scars on them.

Although I had a healthy start in life and a high IQ, to begin with, I spent a lot of time and energy fighting against my potential due to attention deficit hyperactivity disorder (ADHD). Sometimes I wonder how my life and the lives of my wife, kids, and grandkids may have turned out if I had been diagnosed with ADHD when I was younger.

I didn't finish high school because I couldn't concentrate enough to get good grades. I felt my life options were narrowed because I did not complete college. I've wasted millions of dollars that I would have made if I had stuck to the routines that help me manage my ADHD when I mess up a few times. My wealth has fluctuated between the seven figures and negative numbers several times.

My mom always backed me up, told me I could do anything, and helped me feel good about myself. If others hadn't pointed me toward self-improvement resources and encouraged me when I stumbled, I can safely say that the outcome of my life would have been much sadder.

Unfortunately, not everyone is as fortunate as I was in having their ADHD undiagnosed. There's no doubt in my mind that, without the help I received, I would now be either incarcerated, an addict, or dead. This is, unfortunately, the case for many children with ADHD who are now going untreated.

Having undiagnosed ADHD cost me a job and several relationships, but at least that's all I lost. I've been in seventeen car wrecks. My business and finances suffered as a result of these mishaps. It's a miracle I didn't get hurt or kill someone.

I've experienced the relief that comes with effective treatment and management of ADHD and the despair that results when it isn't. I wanted to make a difference, so I decided to join the board of the Inattentive ADHD Coalition. I hope to raise awareness about how detrimental it is to go through life undiagnosed with ADHD.

CHAPTER 10. HOW OTHER MEN WITH ADHD HAVE MANAGED THEIR SYMPTOMS TO START LIVING THEIR BEST LIVES

Because of their unique way of thinking, people with ADHD are considered to possess several useful skills. They have more of an abundance of these traits: spontaneity, creativity, energy, intuition, imagination, and invention. Individuals with ADHD might also hyperfocus on topics that particularly pique their interest more than those without the disorder.

Because of their high energy levels and ability to think independently, these people frequently come up with the most novel and insightful ideas.

Many persons with ADHD can successfully channel their impulsivity into constructive forms of expression, such as spontaneity.

Individuals with ADHD do best in careers that harness their natural energy and enthusiasm for doing new things, whether that's through physical activity, imaginative problem-solving, or some other form of creative expression.

Entrepreneur, innovator, artist, interior designer, graphic designer, paramedic, fireman, police officer, teacher, computer programmer, and athlete are just a few vocations that could work well for someone with ADHD.

Albert Einstein

He created the theory of relativity and became the most famous 20th-century scientist. However, as an adult with ADHD, Albert Einstein represented the norm. He was satisfied with his unkempt appearance and had a reputation for being forgetful. In many ways, he was a law unto himself. After his death, his brain was removed and put in a separate location to be researched.

Sir Richard Branson

British business magnate Sir Richard Branson. He has set up his space exploration corporation and owns an island, making him a powerful figure. His abilities allow him to make significant progress in any endeavor he undertakes.

John F. Kennedy

Before becoming the 35th President of the United States, despite having ADHD, he served in both the House of Representatives and the Senate. As a result, he was more widely covered by the press than either pop artists or Hollywood actors. Despite numerous external hurdles, he was able to secure victories like the Nuclear Test-Ban Treaty.

Will Smith

Despite having ADHD, the "Fresh Prince of Bel-Air" has accomplished a great deal, including writing one of the finest sitcoms ever and releasing successful albums as both an actor and a rapper. According to Newsweek, he is Hollywood's most influential actor. In addition, he enjoys both chess and playing video games.

Jim Carrey

Over two decades, Jim Carrey has been the comedic face of Hollywood. Unfortunately, his inability to control his hyperactive behavior indicates a severe attention deficit hyperactivity disorder. Nevertheless, he's been in some of the funniest films ever made. Treatment for ADHD seems to be helping him.

Adam Levine

Maroon 5's lead vocalist Adam Levine has been open about his struggles with attention deficit hyperactivity disorder (ADHD) in an interview with ADDitute Magazine. He went on to talk about the challenges he faces as an adult songwriter and in the recording studio. He sought medical attention and was informed that what had plagued him since boyhood was still there in his adult life.

Michael Jordan

Success in business and as the owner of the NBA's Charlotte Hornets followed his rise to the top of the basketball world. A hallmark of his disease is an insatiable need to plan his next action. There's an "Air Jordan" emblem on the tail of his jet, which he proudly owns.

Justin Timberlake

JT was unstoppable on the Billboard charts for a long time, and he ended up winning nine Grammys. Then, his "ADD combined with OCD" diagnosis was revealed in an interview with collider.com. Since then, he's established himself as an actor and businessman.

Michael Phelps

When it comes to sports, Michael Phelps is undoubtedly a legend. Phelps has ADHD and attributes much of his success to it, which is why he has won more Olympic gold than anyone else. The Michael Phelps Foundation he established works to expand swimming as a sport and encourage people to lead healthier lives.

Walt Disney

Walt Disney's simplistic drawings become instantly familiar all across the world. Some of his earlier cartoons are still shown on television 50 years after his death. But, amazingly, for someone with ADHD, he originally voiced his most well-known character, Mickey Mouse.

David Neeleman

Does ADHD preclude a person from becoming a highly successful airline CEO? If you don't believe me, ask JetBlue's original CEO, David Neeleman. According to Neeleman, "if given a choice between being normal and keeping my ADD, I would choose my ADD."
I'm scared to use drugs because I'll blow a fuse and end up like everyone else.

This prosperous businessman refuses to treat his disease with medication because he worries about the long-term consequences. Instead, he thinks his ADHD is a big reason for his success.

Many people on board the plane are relieved to hear that Neeleman didn't take the drug. JetBlue Airways wouldn't exist today if he didn't go ahead with the idea. When establishing his airline, Neeleman took great delight in being innovative.

He argues that while ADHD is associated with several negative traits, like disorganization, procrastination, and an inability to focus, it is also associated with creativity and a willingness to take chances.

With confidence, Neeleman declared to the New York media, "We want to be New York's new low-fare, hometown airline." But, coming from a Utah native and Mormon of the third generation, his remarks could be seen as either naive confidence or extraordinary chutzpah.

Neeleman revolutionized air travel by adding features like live in-flight television and outstanding customer service, despite widespread criticism from everyone from venture capitalists who passed on participating in the startup airline to the press.

When Neeleman's teachers failed to recognize their strengths, his parents reminded him of her. "I can take a large amount of information and simplify it so that you can understand it. An entire business plagued by issues inspires me to ask, "How can I do this better?" My hyperactive, inattentive mind constantly looks for more efficient methods.

Neeleman hasn't had the same level of success in his personal life. My family wants me to pay attention to just one item at a time, and my wife often has trouble understanding what I'm thinking. So I'm having a hard time with it.

When I'm feeling down, it's hard for me to perform even the most routine tasks. However, in comparison to paying the electric bill, fleet planning for a fleet of twenty aircraft is a breeze for me.

Neeleman does make an effort to control his thoughts. At work, he teams up with experts in many facets of the company's operations. He explains that he has an assistant who helps him keep a schedule and write letters. From day to day, I have no idea what I'm doing.

So that he doesn't misplace his wallet or keys, he always puts them in the same spot at home. In addition, he uses a Casio DataBank watch, which allows him to quickly jot down notes like meeting times or new ideas as they come to him.

He acknowledges the costs of not treating his ADHD but argues, "Life is full of trade-offs."

What's his counsel for those with attention deficit hyperactivity disorder? Please don't give up hope, he urges; instead, focus on the benefits of having ADHD. Never give up.

Paul Orfalea

He was a lousy student throughout his academic career, failing second grade, earning low grades in high school, and barely scraping by in college. Orfalea has dyslexia and has "ADHD to the fullest," yet he still pursued her dream of being an entrepreneur. Contrarily, it inspired the red-haired, curly-haired executive, better known by his nickname Kinko, to go above and beyond.

In 1970, while Orfalea was still a student at UC Santa Barbara, he had the idea for what would become Kinko's. When he went to the library, he saw a long queue of people waiting to use the photocopy for 10 cents a page.

He reasoned that he could offer the service at a lower price. So Orfalea took out a $5,000 loan and launched the first Kinko's in a renovated hamburger stand near the university. There was just one lone Xerox machine in the room. The success of his copying enterprise led to its acquisition by FedEx.

Orfalea, reflecting on his career, argues that he could seize opportunities because he could " live in the moment" due to his learning condition. The ADHD mind is curious. Seeing is believing, as the saying goes. What others say is accepted by your ears. Over time, I've learned to put faith in my sight.

And so, when consumers started coming in hoping to utilize a computer rather than copy documents, Orfalea saw an opening. He introduced computers to Kinko, which led to its expansion. This resulted in the company gaining the patronage of many self-employed people and owners of small businesses.

He had the ideal mindset for running a business, thanks to his ADHD. But, he admits, "I never spent much time in my workplace since I tended to wander." I was tasked with traveling from store to store and noting the positive practices I encountered.

I would not have found all those great ideas to grow the company if I had stayed at my office all the time. The idea for a 24-hour Kinko's came from the regulars at his shop.

Orfalea states, "I can't fix a machine, and I can't write a letter." But, because of my ADHD, I'm not easily distracted by minor things, which is one of my greatest strengths. I have competent people do that for me.

Orfalea, reflecting on his schooling, thinks schools must accommodate students with varying learning styles to ensure no student falls through the cracks.

According to Orfalea, "No Child Left Behind" would have kept him in third grade because of his poor spelling skills: "If No Child Left Behind had been around while I was in school, I would still be in third grade."

Alan M. Meckler

Meckler claims that his strengths as an entrepreneur stem from his inability to focus, read charts, and understand legal documents. And my impatience made me jump right to the point. After years of academic difficulty as a child, he was diagnosed with dyslexia.

Meckler, who struggled on exams due to his tendency to daydream in class, reflects, "I used to daydream in class a lot. When I couldn't think of the solution immediately, I didn't have the patience to keep working on it. When he was younger, arithmetic (or "math block") was his major stumbling block.

Though he struggled with numbers, he overcame his disabilities and became successful. He claims that he could learn the most important information from a presentation simply by listening to high school and college teachers, while most other students took copious notes.

This is a business skill that I have honed through time. So instead of becoming bogged down, I can zero in on what's most crucial.

Meckler earned a reputation for short meetings at Jupitermedia, the company he formerly led. If you can't explain it in a few words, he says, it probably isn't a good plan.

Meckler adds, "Keep things simple, stupid." Because of his ability to "listen to them, not read about them," he could anticipate emerging business opportunities and seize them before his competitors did.

"I saw the Internet as a business possibility three or four years before anyone else," he claims. So I launched a weekly reporting service covering Internet growth, which became a magazine and is now a trade show.

Between 1994 and 1999, Internet World grew unprecedentedly, becoming one of the most prominent trade shows of all time.

Meckler works in an industry that produces mountains of data, but he has to rely on his coworkers to help him make sense of all the charts, diagrams, and other visual aids. For example, he says I can make sense of basic bar graphs. But, if there are more than two lines on the chart, I lose track of everything.

"I'll go to my chief financial officer and say, 'walk me through this,'" he said, seeking guidance on making sense of economic statistics. If I'm familiar with the subject, I'll be able to understand it immediately; otherwise, I'll be lost. The same goes for balancing his checkbook, which he likewise never does.

In doing so, he is reminded of his childhood, his love of baseball, and his struggles with learning. There were three baseball clubs in New York in the '50s, so young Meckler had enough data to analyze. Thanks to those numbers, he overcame his fear of mathematics.

Those numbers "would be devoured by me," he says. So instead, I taught myself thirds, averaging out, calculating earned run averages in baseball, and mastered the stats. Then he opens up about his struggles with division, saying, "I still have difficulty if you tell me to divide; I can't figure out the numerator or the denominator; I have to look back and think of baseball statistics to help me."

Charles Schwab

Schwab came from a low-income family in a rural area outside Sacramento, and he had to work hard to graduate from Stanford and get a position at a little brokerage firm. So the guy who would build the fourth-largest brokerage firm in the United States started with humble beginnings.

It wasn't until his son was diagnosed with dyslexia that he learned his son had the learning issue. But he knew he needed to put in far more effort than his classmates. He excelled. As a result, he math and science but

Eventually, Schwab overcame dyslexia thanks to his "fairly competent kid" status and "quite extroverted demeanor," as he explained to Fortune Small Business. I had no trouble talking to my teachers and always had many questions for them. That's probably why my professors like me so much. They'd say things like, "Wow, Chuck puts in a lot of effort." We have to raise his grade from C to B.

Because of the challenges he faced due to his learning condition, he became an entrepreneur. He learned humility as a result. No matter how much you think you've accomplished, you can never be sure. That's great inspiration right there. Because of it, he has been able to advance in his job in ways he never thought imaginable.

I knew I was good with numbers even though I had trouble reading," he adds. "I played to my talents and made a career out of my interest in statistics and economics."

He follows in the footsteps of economist Diane Swonk by declaring, "I found something I was brilliant at and grew passionate about." Beyond reading proficiency, I learned that a wide variety of skills and talents are essential for a top executive.

Character, morals, communications skills, persistence, analytical abilities, and interpersonal skills. Such qualities are essential for leaders. I possess a few of those skills, and I'm fortunate to collaborate with many talented people.

The quality of generosity is another one of his strengths. Schwab's kid was diagnosed with dyslexia, and the businessman and his wife, Helen, decided to lend a hand to other families in similar situations. As a result, the Schwab Foundation was established to address the overwhelming number of concerns that arise when a kid is experiencing academic difficulties.

Like many other successful CEOs, Schwab recognizes the importance of teamwork. He says a group of "strong people around me" deals with the "day-to-day planning and organizing," he says. They have taught me how to streamline my paperwork and reduce the amount of reading I have to do.

There isn't much of a difference between this and the experience of most persons in executive positions in major organizations. To get things done, you need a dedicated group of people.

If Schwab could advise those who also struggle with learning disabilities like ADHD or dyslexia, what would he say?

What you're good at should be your primary focus; hone in on it, and give it double the effort you normally would. Making the most of one's circumstances is a goal all humanity shares. Think about what you're good at. Please do not be reluctant to accept assistance or to admit that you require it. See where that advice led Schwab.

Stephen Ilyas

I entered the world on August 1, 1977, between 6 and 7. I arrived a full month before my due date. In retrospect, this is one of the rare instances in which I arrived early.

I had no say in the matter, but I also had no say in many other situations that demanded my prompt presence. It appeared that I lacked the necessary discipline in time management, and while my accomplishments have thus far been largely disregarded, I have constantly and notably failed to arrive on time.

Maybe I was like a lot of kids my age. My mom was a stay-at-home mom while my dad worked out of the house. My family and I lived in a static caravan in a wooded area. Around an oval green were other oblong houses, and beyond our caravan, the wood rose steeply to an unfamiliar location. I once took a chance and climbed the hillside trail near these woods to see what was beyond.

Trees spoke to me, and I knew right then that I was destined for a life of exploration.

The Desire To Know And Ask Questions

When I was in school, I found that Art and English were the most stimulating for my creative spirit—reading, writing, and drawing all formed vivid scenes in my mind. Other classes just seemed boring to me. I used to be the kid who constantly bugged adults with "Why?" when they were supposed just to let me learn my lesson.

When I started something deemed disrespectful, whatever that may imply, I was often met with responses intended as punishments. I was supposed to listen and absorb, but I was never very good at those things.

After graduating college in 1993, I made a vow to never again put on a tie except in two specific situations: (a) if a prospective employer specifically requested one or (b) if a solicitor strongly advised it. While I've never considered option B, I bought a tie on one of my many spur-of-the-moment shopping visits and wore it once (just for fun).

ADHD And The Workplace

Now that I was ready to enter the workforce, I quickly saw how few opportunities were available. Even in Art and Design, I only managed a C; my best GCSE score was a D in English. So following that decision, I spent the next thirteen years building and refining my resume.

I began my career as an apprentice sign maker, and a college printing course that had initially piqued my curiosity quickly became tedious. Nevertheless, I have zero regrets about leaving.

I have experience working in various settings, including as a warehouse worker, a food factory worker, a ventilation pipe installer, and a nightclub cleaner. Previously, I worked as a "telesales executive." Extremely boring, yet the bills had to be paid.

Some work experiences were really enjoyable. For example, I helped load stage sets, instruments, and sound and lighting equipment at a haulage company specializing in transporting musical productions on tour. AC/DC was my very first employer. At one point, I worked for the Iron Maiden Fan Club and the Rolling Stones and went around Europe with both organizations.
When I finished school, I became a guitar technician and tour manager for a band that took me all around England and Ireland. In addition, I spent time building stages and other scenery for various theater productions.

While working in live theater, I had the opportunity to run Dobbin, the animatronic puppet horse, for a performance of Dr. Doolittle while Phillip Schofield affixed glasses to the horse's head. So naturally, I decided then and there that I would become a puppeteer...

Lost Satellite

While some seem naturally drawn to the pursuits that excite them, I spent most of my early adult years in perpetual motion, unsure of where I was headed. I felt like a satellite without any coordination to guide me.

I had been employed at a small, locally-owned clothes shop in Norwich and had been persuaded to join a branch in Glasgow... The answer is obvious: I went through my glam semi-transvestite phase after being offered a job at an "alternative" clothing store after a year. I settled on entering the hairdressing industry. I packed and headed back to good old Norwich...

Since I was unemployed and had any relevant skills, I had zero confidence and zero optimism. I couldn't understand why I was having so much trouble getting started. Likewise, my thoughts and body seemed to be in a constant state of motion. So there goes another broken heart.

Still another unpaid bill. Yet another debt collector called about that unpaid cell phone bill, that Open University loan for that programming course, that overdraft at the bank, etc.
Over time, these bills would be paid, and the process would begin again. Oh no, not again! And I still don't know how to handle my finances. So why do I get so giddy about this? To what end am I perpetually distracted? Why can't I relax?

However, I did frequently switch to other activities. I never stopped drawing, sketching, and painting in my spare time—nearly compulsive behavior. In a bar, I connected with a man who was a friend of a friend. He patiently endured my nonstop babbling and then offered wise counsel. He was an undergraduate at the time and has since earned a Ph.D. in Organic Chemistry. When it comes to friendship, we haven't changed a bit:

"Man, why don't you devote yourself to doing art? You have a creative mind.Am I?

My exposure to the ideas of famous philosophers, artists, writers, and musicians increased as I spent more time with him and his lovely partner, who also attended university. So what made me think I belonged at this exclusive club of the rich and the smart?

In 2007, I applied to Norwich University College of the Arts computer game design program and attended an interview where I presented a portfolio of my drawings. Naturally, I saw right then that a career in video game design was where my interests lay.

It was a terrible interview. My standard response to every inquiry was, "No, I have not done that." Though I went home feeling discouraged, I did as my interviewer suggested and started looking for a college course that would help me get into university and onto the course that was a good fit for my skills and interests.

Stay Focused, Stay Focused, Stay Focused!

When Brenda Unwin, who interviewed me at the last minute, informed me that several of my drawings showed great competence and that she would be glad to award me a spot on the Access to Higher Education course, I almost burst into tears. Never in my life have I felt such overwhelming joy.

In between dumping off my paintings (one of which was still wet) at the end-of-year show and using the facilities, of course. When I returned, the painting was still wet, but there was a letter saying the principal had bought it for the school.

That seemed impossible to me. A friend with a Ph.D. came to see the show and bought a self-portrait. I had it professionally framed, and now it proudly hangs in their living room.

I continued my education and enjoyed the best time of my life in college. And when things became rough, I was treated with respect and compassion as an adult. Still, I couldn't stop jumping from one thing to the next; however, this might be an asset throughout the creative process.

Despite a decent first year of schooling, my second-year grades dropped significantly due largely to the increased emphasis on independent study. My tutor said it was not unusual as we entered the third, final, and crucial year. It would help if you focused very hard.

The start of my third year found me in the difficult position of being unable to think coherently about anything. Ideas, possibilities, and uncertainty flooded my head. Why do I feel so confused when I have so much information? Those weeks of awkward fear have been preserved in a sketchbook I have kept. Graduation ceremony time quickly approached.

I had won a prize for my paintings, and the university and the late actor Sir John Hurt had purchased pieces for permanent collections. The man communicated with me. The inverted order is incorrect.

While I was being interviewed about my impressive graduation exhibition, my tutor Brenda came to take a look. This time, I let the tears come freely. I was and am very appreciative. I am indebted to you for a great deal. I'm grateful that strangers took the time to hear me out and direct me to safety.

However, having a degree didn't help me get a job. So, for the next four years, I actively pursued my painting career, holding exhibitions in London (at two major art fairs), Bath, Cambridge, and Norwich. In addition, I cleaned a bar and a house to make ends meet so I could pursue my artistic interests.

I made it through some hard patches thanks to the support of friends and, later, a wife who shared my values and cared about me. Of course, I appreciated the help, but I was still annoyed. Despite knowing what I wanted, wanted, and needed to achieve, I couldn't figure out why I couldn't do them. I was constantly falling. I made numerous attempts at focusing, acting professionally, etc.

My First NHS Appointment

As 2015 progressed, I became increasingly frustrated. Tossing my phone around like a ragdoll, frivolously spending money, and being distracted from my goals were finally too much. Then, after making an appointment with the National Health Service's (NHS) psychiatry department, I was diagnosed with bipolar disorder. Thus, I went and educated myself on the subject.

Some of the symptoms fit my experiences, and I had thought about suicide frequently and almost carried it out in 2014. However, I never experienced regular lows and highs, so I wasn't certain that I had cyclothymia, a moderate type of Bipolar.

There is no one more encouraging than my wife. She is, in fact, very encouraging to anybody she meets. My uniqueness has always stood out to her, but she also recognizes that this is what makes me so intriguing and has done so since the day we first met. The fact that she intentionally and openly chooses me as her husband is still incomprehensible to me.

There was a major rift between us because I consistently failed to act appropriately, manage finances responsibly, and follow through on my commitments. And it wasn't simply my moods, either; something else was at play. I am pursuing a master's degree in art history and theory at Essex.

Something was off the whole time I was in school. The material offered piques my attention. I find myself intrigued by the points raised. In particular, I'm curious about the school's demographic makeup. The fact that I am frequently a minority viewpoint is something I find incredibly intriguing. The truth of being ignorant is something that fascinates me much.

Research is something I'd like to learn more about. It's a hobby of mine that I enjoy. Although I enjoy reading, I usually have to skim the next several paragraphs. Why do I have such difficulty focusing on things that truly pique my interest? I don't understand why I feel so out of place in a room full of bright, creative minds.

Because of this, I tried to confront my problems and learn the origins of my flaky character. Then, I was acutely aware of my incapacity to engage in activities that brought me joy and satisfaction consciously. But what could I do?

I knew I had not voluntarily signed up for a lifetime of hardship. Instability in my finances is not something I voluntarily choose. I didn't seek out a job that didn't allow me to pursue my passions.

In other words, I want to follow my desires. If I weren't forbidden, I'd ask, "Why can't I?" I didn't understand what was wrong with my mind. Then I came across an article, and suddenly everything made sense… The next step was to investigate whether or not having ADHD was a possibility for me.

I suggested it to my GP. In contrast to cyclothymia, which I was also familiar with, all of the symptoms described in the literature seemed to reflect my experience. I was familiar with the arrangement but had never attempted to paint it. It was a good match for the body. It became more familiar to me as I read on. They all fit, and not just some of them.

The National Health Service is truly a masterpiece of democratic design. As a result, everyone, regardless of their race, religion, gender identity, or political leanings, has access to quality healthcare in their area.

I am frustrated by how politicians appear to be working to undermine our system. Choosing to prioritize health is not a matter for the political arena. People of questionable moral character are not the only ones entitled to medical care. Yes, money will be needed.

But surely nobody would refuse to put in a few additional cents, or even a pound, to help maintain it. Unfortunately, the NHS cannot promptly offer many forms of mental health care. Unfortunately, it was unable to refer me to a specialized psychiatrist who could diagnose and treat my possible ADHD.

Reports of people taking their own lives because they couldn't get help fast enough are all too common. For example, my sister-in-law, who was 24 years old, tragically committed suicide. She was brilliant, hilarious, and a pleasure to be around, but her mental health issues were insurmountable.
Now that her estate is settled, my wife has some extra cash and has recommended we use it to determine what my mind is up to, turning our sorrow into something constructive. Psychiatry-UK LLP is a CQC-accredited online psychiatry service, and I decided to schedule an appointment with them.

Why the National Health Service doesn't cover their service is a mystery to me. I had my doubts. The question, "Are these persons qualified?" ' Seriously, what do psychiatric professionals know? After reading some of the expert profiles on the internet, I realized I was in over my head and had to seek help.

One morning, my wife and I watched a webinar where Dr. Andy Montgomery discussed ADHD in adults, including its symptoms, causes, effects, and whether or not general practitioners could recognize a patient with the disorder.

Understanding What Is Meant By "Hyperfocus"

Dr. Montgomery's slide about high-achieving students with ADHD who went on to college but struggled due to the increased demands of higher education caught my interest.

These people said, "I can't do this, not because I don't have the ability, I do, but because I can't keep up with speed, I can't read the material without getting distracted, I can't focus without a distraction."

He described a state of hyperfocus, in which one is so absorbed in an activity that nothing else registers. For example, I remember spending six weeks on a single essay, writing at least eight thousand main text words and another two thousand in notes and citations.

I just kept going. The essay I produced in 13 hours the day before the deadline and the one I spent days on both earned the same grade. Such an approach to work is inefficient at best.

I scheduled a meeting with the first person who could see me and conversed with Dr. Stephen Ilyas a few days later. It was refreshing to have a conversation with a level-headed expert. He listened attentively, and I felt better afterward. Next, he contacted my dad and mom to obtain their perspectives, and a few days later, I got the news.

In the first week of April 2017, I was diagnosed with attention deficit hyperactivity disorder. Medicine has been recommended for me. There was a sense of relief but also of loss. Have I been squandering the past two decades? Perhaps. When I think of what I could have done if… How would my relationship with my mom be if... What if I asked...?

It's natural to have these thoughts. However, the past is the past, and dwelling on missed opportunities is pointless. Possibilities exist for everyone, but I finally feel like I can realize mine.

Although I still have some difficulties after taking my medication, they are now limited to reading challenging materials, and I am scheduled to see a doctor soon to determine whether or not I suffer from visual stress, a condition shared by many people with ADHD. The diagnosis has helped me gain some insight into who I am.

Medication allows me to block out the background noises...

My prescription to help me concentrate allows me to explore Ph.D. programs. However, I don't have to, and it would be silly to take medication when I plan to relax at the beach, prepare a meal for friends, hike in the woods, or do anything else that doesn't require intense focus.

Personal opinion: I love having ADHD. People tend to laugh at me because I do many ridiculous things. I like that a lot. However, when it results in negative outcomes, ADHD is a concern. A number of the activities that society expects of you cannot do while you are in this state. As a result of the condition, some things are much better for society.

My diagnosis and subsequent prescription have put me in a position to make strategic use of ADHD. In graduating from college, I will be just as stuck with few options as I was after high school. Now that I'm focusing on what I enjoy, my ADHD has less impact on the areas where it isn't necessary.

Ren

First, my best friend called me to tell me that her son, with whom I am very close, had been diagnosed with attention deficit hyperactivity disorder (ADHD). After we had all finished crying and processing the implications of his diagnosis, I pledged to be there for them.

My friend's growing understanding of ADHD led me to wonder if a more fundamental issue was at the root of my difficulties in succeeding. Perhaps I wasn't completely unmotivated, insane, and dim-witted.

Even though I was aware of my intelligence, I could not maintain interest in or focus on any given task for an extended period. My gAs a result, models have been a poor ref. Having a full-time job has always been stressful and melancholy for me.

Anxiety and worry arose from the weight of the burdensome responsibilities. And my feelings were in charge of me. When things were going well, I felt like the world was made of sunshine and lollipops, but even the smallest setback would send me into a tailspin of rage and self-loathing.

The day I learned I had attention deficit hyperactivity disorder was the day I finally started to believe in myself and my abilities.

I participated in a program that would have prepared me for life after high school two years after my diagnosis because I was curious about what life could have been like for me had I been diagnosed as a youngster and because I needed reassurance that I wasn't an idiot.

My parents, siblings, and I were pleased with how I handled my course workload, time commitments, exams, and emotional and mental well-being. In 2021, after I finish my degree in environmental science, I will finally be able to pursue my passion.

My condition has improved thanks to medication, but I am still not completely healthy. Whenever my medication stops working, which is usually around bedtime, I am again plagued by my initial symptoms. Even now, I can't handle a lot of noise and commotion all at once.

I still forget what I'm saying, get depressed and anxious, and have trouble understanding the point of queries. Even with medication, which is said to help kids with ADHD complete assignments in a weekend, I still need at least two weeks to complete a two thousand-word paper.

My diagnosis has boosted my sense of self-worth and confidence, allowing me to live a happier, more secure, and more fulfilled life.

Jo

My ADHD diagnosis came at the age of 28. I had been having trouble learning new processes at work, and after watching the symptoms listed on TV, I went to see my doctor to receive a referral. Since he insisted there was no such thing as ADHD, I had to insist on a referral. He looked for a psychiatrist on Google, and I brought my school records and a friend to meet with him.

When I finally got a diagnosis, I felt so much better. My whole life, I had battled with problems nobody else ever had. I had been called lazy and had begun to accept the epithet as true about myself. But I was also sad because perhaps if I had been diagnosed sooner, things wouldn't have been so difficult for me. Would I have been more successful if I had tried?

My perception of my flaws shifted, and I gained a newfound appreciation for my strengths due to my diagnosis. Once I found the right resources to help me, I became more compassionate toward myself and inspired to improve the areas where I'd previously been inadequate.

After discussing drug options with me, my psychiatrist recommended me to a psychologist-led support group. This method greatly enhanced my ability to plan, concentrate, problem-solve, and maintain momentum.

As a bonus, I can focus on the task, eliminate distractions, and increase my output. It helps me concentrate, but the negative side effects mean I only use it sometimes.

Chris

At 43, I was diagnosed with the same diagnosis as my 16-year-old daughter. I had spent the previous six months (while waiting for my psychiatrist appointment) deliberating between the ideas that I had and did not have attention deficit hyperactivity disorder (ADHD).

My psychiatrist recommended Ritalin, and I'm still experimenting with my optimal dosage and administration schedule. Finding an effective dosage while minimizing side effects can be tricky.

However, ever since I started taking Ritalin, everything has become a lot less difficult. I used to, for instance:

- It gave me the impression that I was viewing an outdated TV with plenty of static. I could make out the image and some of the dialogue, but it took a lot of effort and focus. However, I feel like the image has been adjusted to perfection, and I can finally hear and see it clearly without strain.

- Put off work till the last minute. But, "getting started" was a major challenge for me. I was at a loss as to how to initiate difficult tasks. In addition, I had a hard time learning to prioritize my work.

  My mind was racing with random ideas, and sustained mental effort left me physically and emotionally exhausted.

  When I came home, I was too tired to do anything and couldn't recall what I had intended to do that night. I was just a couch potato. I used to have trouble concentrating, but ever since I started taking Ritalin, I've been able to plan and get things done.

  It's convenient because I can go straight to my workplace and go to work. As a result, I've gained a lot of strength and energy and no longer collapsed at the end of the day.

- This resonates with me as someone who has always considered themselves rather shy and has struggled with anxiety (including stomach problems, heart racing, a "thumping" heart rate, etc.). As a result, I used to avoid either or not spending much time at huge social gatherings.

  But ever since I began taking Ritalin, my anxiety has completely vanished. I've gained a lot of confidence in social situations, and I look forward to going to work now.

It's still early, but the diagnosis and treatment seem to be helping me quite a little. The unknowns of the future intrigue me.

Michael

Until around three years ago, I considered myself a fully functional human.

Usually, I'm the type to give the impression that I'm attentive when, in reality, my mind is wandering, thinking about everything and everything that catches my eye at the moment.

The type of person who stays up until 3 am thinking about what they want to do tomorrow.

A person who, although competent in any endeavor they set their mind to (if they could control their mind), cannot remain in one line of work for more than a few years. And the person who starts a project, then another, then another, and then... forgets what they were working on before.

I used to believe everybody desperately sought the limelight at whatever cost. "Just look at all the adoration they have for me!" (Despite my tendency to be too dominant and to complete other people's thoughts and sentences).

'Wow! I pray this is how things always are! So why should I change anything? My life is functioning in some wacky, chaotic fashion, and I'm perfectly content with bluffing my way through it. Until:

- The lack of sleep and striving to maintain order caused fatigue.

- Whenever I tried to focus, my eyesight blurred.

- Communication with loved ones and strangers alike became increasingly difficult for me.

- I began having problems with my ability to remember things in the short term.

- Due to my extreme sensitivity, I frequently found myself losing my temper.

Undiagnosed Attention Deficit Hyperactivity Disorder was to blame. Fortunately, I could schedule an appointment with a psychiatrist, who quickly diagnosed me with the disease and put me on medication (stimulant treatment).

Despite the ups and downs of readjusting to life without constant mental cloudiness and coming to terms with the fact that I need medication to help me think more clearly, I can now get my life back on track and do all that needs doing without wearing myself out.

Consequently, although I accept my ADHD diagnosis and recognize that I am completely typical for someone with the disorder, I do not feel "there" yet. Nonetheless, I am confident that I am making progress correctly. When I start to feel discouraged about how tough it is to keep pushing on, my wife, who has been my rock through this ordeal, thankfully reminds me of how far I have come and how much I have accomplished since my diagnosis.

Clinton

Getting an ADHD diagnosis at age 24 was a huge weight off my shoulders. I was a restless kid who struggled to focus in class and never quite felt like I "fit in." But then, all the pieces of the puzzle suddenly fit together. It all made perfect sense.

As far back as I can remember, I've suspected that I have attention deficit hyperactivity disorder. My struggle to find the proper doctor, get the right diagnosis, and get the right advice was complicated and time-consuming because I also suffer from Anxiety, Depression, OCD, Tourette's Syndrome, and Post-Traumatic Stress Disorder.

Now that I am medicated for my ADHD, I cannot do anything without it. It helps me feel strong and capable of getting through each day.

Despite the difficulties of ADHD, I am pleased to report that I have a happy, fulfilling life. Because I refuse to allow hyperactivity/attention deficit hyperactivity disorder (ADHD) to define me, I stand out from the crowd; it's a special element of who I am.

Brian Scudamore

At the age of 18, Brian Scudamore entered the so-called "junk business" as a means to fund his education. While waiting at a McDonald's drive-through, he observed a pickup truck emptying garbage cans, and that's when the idea hit him.

Scudamore purchased a truck for his new business and dubbed his company the Rubbish Boys. He decided at 23 that education wasn't for him and instead focused on his business.
He finally realized that learning how to operate a business effectively required running one. Scudamore currently serves as the chief executive officer of O2E Brands, a franchisor that operates under four brands: 1-800-GOT-JUNK?, Wow 1 Day Painting, You Move Me, and Shack Shine.

Scudamore is the epitome of the phrases "distracted, high-energy, and impetuous." Yet, Scudamore claims that knowing his strengths and weaknesses has helped him tremendously in his battle to keep his symptoms under control.

When running the day-to-day operations of his business, he is less than stellar, but he is excellent at coming up with big ideas and producing vision. Rather than trying to accomplish everything alone, he employs a "two-in-the-box" strategy in which he and his chief operating officer (COO) work together to make the company's vision a reality.

A lot of effort is required to control ADHD. Scudamore says, "Over the years, I had to build tools and tactics to get something done quickly and efficiently." He's realized that keeping active helps him concentrate more.

Moving around between offices helps him maintain focus for longer periods. For example, he uses the constant hum of a coffee shop to focus his CEO's mind.

Matt Curry

Seventh-grader Matt Curry was diagnosed with attention deficit hyperactivity disorder in 1978. After a year on Ritalin, his parents and physicians agreed to wean him off. That was encouraging news for Curry, who previously believed he needed medication to function well with ADHD.
After graduating from college, Curry gained experience in the automobile industry by working for several stores, where he successfully increased sales and profits. From a single location, he expanded into one of the largest independent auto-repair businesses in the Greater Washington, D.C. area, with ten locations.

Curry published the book The A.D.D. Entrepreneur to aid other business owners; he also offers consulting services to those who want to replicate his success.

According to Curry, his hyperactivity disorder is his greatest asset. To paraphrase, "It's because of it, not despite it, that I've been successful." Each day, he employs certain methods for channeling his boundless enthusiasm and inventiveness.

When he has too many thoughts to keep track of, he writes them down on a whiteboard and then prioritizes them into "three things I need to do." Then, what he wants, how he plans to accomplish it, and why he plans to accomplish it are all dissected into a vision, game plan, and message.

When his thoughts start to run, he strolls into the car or heads to his office to meditate until he can collect his thoughts. It depends on the situation; sometimes Curry works best in a group setting, where he can bounce ideas off of people, and sometimes he works best alone, where he can focus on his thoughts.

If you've been diagnosed with ADHD, Curry says you should accept it. Place yourself in winning scenarios, he advises. People with ADHD tend to excel in business. There's a chance you would thrive in a helping profession, such as social work. Make the most of your abilities and figure out your route in life.

Peter Shankman

Peter Shankman, frequently sent to the principal's office for talking too much in class, must feel pretty good about himself now that he is in high demand as a professional speaker. In addition, he is sought as an expert in many fields, including customer service, marketing, social media, and more.

Shankman was raised in New York City, where he resides with his wife and two-year-old daughter. A burning need to disprove the notion that he was a "slow learner," as his professors had claimed, drove him to rise from "class clown" to respected corporate consultant, author, and entrepreneur.

Shankman diligently pursued his bachelor's degree in journalism and photojournalism at Boston University. Help a Reporter Out (HARO) and The Geek Factory, a social media, marketing, and PR strategy agency based in New York City, are his namesakes.

Until his late twenties, Shankman claims he rarely exercised beyond jogging to McDonald's to pick up Big Macs and to the grocery store to pick up packs of smokes. He is now a licensed skydiver, runner, and Ironman finisher who uses exercise as a substitute for conventional ADHD medicine.

As a result of his difficult upbringing (he had dyslexia and was ridiculed at school for a spell), he feels compelled to reassure children that better days are ahead. As a result, he frequently addresses students and teachers in New York City high schools on the issue of attention deficit hyperactivity disorder.

Despite being prescribed medication for ADHD in his late twenties, Shankman chooses not to take any. As he puts it, "my level of dopamine when I go skydiving or for a long run is the same as taking Ritalin or Adderall." Skydiving, Shankman says, gives him perspective. "It helps me concentrate and think more clearly."

Shankman admits that before he learned to control his ADHD, "I constantly delayed until the last minute [to complete anything], or I'd forget stuff." Finally, he's figured out how to use this strategy of waiting until the end to his benefit.

The standard time allotted by my publisher for me to complete a book draft is six months. Typically, I don't do anything until the last week of the month. I get a ticket to Tokyo and compose chapters 1–5 on the plane there, then chapters 6–10 on the journey back. That's the only productive method I've ever encountered.

Shankman has found that he is most productive at home with his two-year-old daughter when he puts away his devices. She is the primary center of my attention in most of my waking hours, and our conversations take up most of my time. Just taking things as they come is what I like to do.

Shankman says he "stops at the door and I take 10 long, deep breaths" before he enters his home with his wife and children. It calms me down and helps me approach the situation with an open mind.

Shankman does not consider his ADHD to be an issue. What you have is not a sickness; rather, it is a blessing. You'll need to figure out how to handle it.

We have a greater capacity for rapid thought and processing than the average person, and this is true whether or not we choose to alter our brain chemistry with drugs or merely by engaging in a brief bout of vigorous exercise. That's fantastic, and it's something we should embrace.

Shane Perrault

Shane Perrault, a psychologist, had an early introduction to attention deficit hyperactivity disorder (ADHD), though he didn't realize it at the time. Perrault's academic performance was either excellent or bad.

"History education was a haze of information that I struggled to make sense of. Soon I felt completely overrun," he admits.

Perrault's parents cared deeply for him, but his academic performance disheartened them. Moreover, they had no idea what was wrong with their bright boy.

The breakthrough occurred during an eleventh-grade course on religions other than Western ones. The teacher introduced movies and role-play into the classroom to appeal to Perrault's kinesthetic learning approach.

He brought it to life, as Perrault puts it. "I figured out that education was enjoyable for me but that my learning process was unique. So I enrolled in courses such as public speaking and debate piqued my interest.

Through college, Perrault got by on his superior intelligence and the subjects that piqued his curiosity. However, this strategy was useless in graduate school because there was too much work. This prompted Perrault to create a set of study techniques tailored to the needs of those with attention deficit hyperactivity disorder.

In 40- to 50-minute study sessions, he would take 10-minute breaks. Then, for his board examinations, Perrault skated while listening to recorded study material because he found that mobility aided his learning. When I studied that way, I always retained everything I read.

It's no secret that Perrault's ADHD hampered his social skills. Everybody in my hometown cheered for the college team where I grew up. But, he admits, "I was in my universe." If the group is discussing sports and you know nothing about it, you won't win them over.

Perrault first rejected the idea that he had ADHD when it was offered to him by a professor in graduate school. When he first started trying to help me, I didn't recognize it as such. That's when I realized he was trying to ditch me. Finally, his condition was validated through a paper-and-pencil test administered at the university's counseling department.

"I had been trying to understand why I was wired differently than my peers, so [the diagnosis] was a relief. My peers were like sponges at remembering information, but I was terrible at it.

Despite his difficulties with memorization, Perrault was a talented author. If there were negative reviews, I would offer explanations that nobody else would have thought of.

Skating and cycling are only two of the ways that Perrault gets his ADHD under control these days. I'd rather put in 100-150 miles per week on my bike than take medication. I have an endorphin addiction. During this time, Perrault reads up on fascinating authors, such as Carl Jung and Abraham Maslow.

He uses the same techniques he learned in graduate school to stay focused and energized in his professional life, such as conducting marketing activities in a lively setting, such as a coffee shop, instead of at a desk.

Through self-management of his ADHD, he overcame his previous shyness. "As I became more self-aware and effective at managing my ADHD, I began associating with others who excelled in [such settings]. I realized they had unspoken social norms, and when I began to adopt those norms, my social life flourished.

Not only does Perrault run a thriving ADHD clinic, but he is also in demand as a speaker, having recently addressed the Congressional Black Caucus on the Black family. About ADHD, Perrault has spoken to congregations and parent organizations like CHADD.

Perrault believes that ADHD helps him in his professional and entrepreneurial endeavors. I couldn't imagine life without ADHD any more than Superman could imagine life without his cape.

It's helped me connect with others, understand them, and appreciate their good qualities, so I think it's given me some unique skills in dealing with others. Having that skill is crucial for a psychologist.

Dave Farrow

Due to his bad handwriting and spelling, Dave Farrow was considered a slow student in elementary school in Kitchener-Waterloo, Ontario. Today, he holds the Guinness World Record for Greatest Memory on two separate occasions. The notion that I am a slow learner has been bothersome to Farrow. Determined to disprove his teachers, he went out to do so.

Farrow received her ADHD diagnosis when he was 14 years old. He reasoned that there must be some benefit to being in his situation, and he set out to discover what it was. "I had a lot of problems studying in the classroom, but I had a huge desire for learning in general," Farrow adds.

When he was in high school, he would often be found in the school library, immersed in a book on a subject that interested him. He looked at methods like speed-reading and simple visualization to boost his study skills. He used these aids to construct his memory training method in high school.

Farrow, an avid sports fan, pondered whether or not he could benefit from applying interval training, a common method of sport-training, to his mental fitness. To put his theory to the test, he worked feverishly for exactly two minutes and fifty-five seconds using an egg timer.

He decided to try to memorize a huge list of foreign vocabulary terms in that period, which was an extremely challenging job. I would be trying quite hard to accomplish this, though.

His stopwatch beeped, and he paused when it reached zero. It took him about two minutes, but he used that time to do something he enjoyed—like playing video games—to get his thoughts straight. Then he started all over again.

According to Farrow, he avoided distraction and exhaustion by studying in shorter intervals. Farrow's method relies on chemical processes in the brain to analyze data. Farrow argues that overwork leads to a depletion of brain chemicals that aid with concentration.

Short work intervals allowed him to recover more quickly, concentrate more intently, and retain nearly all the information he was exposed to. Rather than waiting for my brain to intervene, I learned to rein in my hyperfocus by stopping myself.

"By the time I mastered these methods, I had become so proficient in my studies that I dropped out of high school to launch my company, Wizardtech Inc., because I was so bored with the pace at which I was being taught."

Farrow taught businesses and individuals how to improve productivity by memorizing information that would otherwise be looked up, reducing wasted time.

Gaining his first Guinness World Record in 1996 for Greatest Memory was a turning point in Farrow's professional life. As a result of his success, he began receiving corporate clients, appearing on television, and collaborating with neuroscientists at McGill University on a pilot study based on The Farrow Memory Training Technique.

Farrow, an "adrenaline junkie," doesn't take medicine for his ADHD or concurrent bipolar disorder; he uses sports instead. "The high I get from resistance training just helps me out."

Farrow's dating life and friendships suffered as a result of her addiction to adrenaline. To find "the one," I had to go through several unsuccessful relationships. He finally tied the knot with Andrea in 2008.

Farrow has found that his unconventional methods have helped him thrive. There is a wide variety of possible identities one can adopt. We have been struck by lightning, and as a result, we are different from everyone else. What's the point in trying to fit in? What's the harm in celebrating your uniqueness?

Maya Bolton

I had to end a call early because I had important business. Even though I was only distracted for a short period, I completely forgot about the call. I had forgotten everything about it until something reminded me the next day.

This sort of disconnection is, sadly, not uncommon for me. For example, as I make my way through the house in the morning, I often find myself reciting reminders to myself, such as "Turn off the iron" or "Keys" (as a slap to the forehead on the way out the door). Likewise, I frequently dash home shortly after getting to the workplace to grab a notebook or file.

My loved ones and coworkers have been understanding and have always just put it down to my "being a little spacey" They would tell me that I make up for my flaws with my many endearing traits. My forgetfulness, though, seemed out of hand as of late.

Ignoring phone calls was becoming increasingly offensive. My chronic procrastination had become clinically significant. My "eye" was also becoming remarkably unreliable in the workplace, where I usually edit documents. Even my manager saw it. After exhausting all my options, I consulted a psychologist for help.

My Doctor's Observation

After hearing my background story, he made an unexpected suggestion: maybe I was hyperactive due to attention deficit hyperactivity disorder (ADHD).

Nonetheless, aren't those who have to ADD typically hyperactive? When in doubt, I questioned. Although I have an attention-deficit/hyperactivity disorder (ADHD), I am not hyperactive; my friends and family will witness this.
This body doesn't budge even though the mind is working at full speed. This was true even more so in my younger years when ADD was typically diagnosed.

There are three subtypes of attention deficit hyperactivity disorder (ADHD), with primarily hyperactive and predominantly inattentive being the most known.

The latter type is characterized by daydreaming and a tendency to tune out during group activities. Subtle symptoms mean they are often misdiagnosed. There are more women than men.

The psychologist speculated that I might have been experiencing ADD type two.

Mixed Reactions

In the following weeks, I encountered widespread skepticism and hostility when discussing ADHD with those in my social circle. "Focus," my coworker advised me. "People living with ADHD have trouble concentrating." (Her assumptions were incorrect. People with ADD are capable of focused attention; it just doesn't last.

A friend told me, "You've got too much on your plate." She made a valid argument. I had a lot of balls in the air at once. Was I just overcommitted?

"Oh, ADD," another person sighed. Isn't that the prevailing chaos right now?
It would appear to be so. The number of ADHD diagnoses has doubled since 1990, and the trend line only appears to be upward. A lot of people seem interested in reading about this. Thus publishers of books on the subject have done well. Vendors sell ADD-pride merchandise like t-shirts and mugs at conventions with themes like "Living the ADDventure," as well as specialized ADD datebooks and coaching services for chronically disorganized people.

Students with ADD in high school and often in college are eligible for extended standardized test periods.

An increase in childhood diagnoses is contributing to the growth. The newly diagnosed do include some adults, though.

In 1990, NIH psychiatrist Alan Zametkin reported findings from positron-emission tomography scans linking ADD with at least one physical sign in the brain: decreased activity in the prefrontal cortex, from where planning and self-control emerge. Moreover, according to the findings of other experts, this condition appears to have a strong genetic component.

Conflicting Viewpoints

The research has not resolved an ongoing controversy over the prevalence of ADD in adults. However, some skeptics argue that psychologists are too hasty in making such diagnoses without adequate research. Nevertheless, several of the newly discovered do meet the psychologist's description of the personality type that could benefit from therapy; even skeptics admit this.

Consequently, I opted for the tougher of the two evaluations. The three-hour session gave me a battery of reading comprehension, memory, and problem-solving exams.
The TOVA (Test of Variability of Attention), which involves seeing an orange square emerge and vanish on a computer screen, was the most annoying.

It would help if you did nothing when a square emerges in the bottom-right corner of the screen. It would help if you pressed the button when it shows above. Not rocket science. Wrong. I tried humming and biting my lip to concentrate, but I still managed to make a shocking number of mistakes.

My early life was littered with warning indications of the disorder. For example, when I was a kid, and I asked my mom a question, she usually wanted to know how long she had to respond.

She anticipated I would give her that blank stare; she understood that I was preoccupied with other things and eager to go on. I was the prototypical student who couldn't focus on what was being taught in class and underachieved.

The doctor and I agreed that my condition was a textbook example of attention deficit hyperactivity disorder (inattentive subtype). I was further persuaded by my reaction when she gave me her view; I cried out of relief that I finally had an explanation for the issues that had been bothering me for so long, as well as anxiety at the ramifications of the diagnosis.

Finally, what comes next? Adults with ADHD can be helped with various workbooks and coaching programs that teach them techniques for improving their concentration and staying on task. In contrast, a low dose of the stimulant medication Ritalin is typically recommended for the underlying focus problem, especially for someone who undertakes a detail-oriented job.

Although I am not qualified to comment on the debates raised about this medicine, especially regarding its usage in minors, I can attest that even a small dose has helped me tremendously. It allows me to maintain an editorial focus for up to four hours.I have a clearer sense of direction and better recall recent events. (I receive all of these advantages with no negative consequences.) In addition, I had a perfect score on the medication section of the TOVA when I retook the test.

Even though I have changed for the better, I still get anxious. I worry that if my coworkers found out about my condition, they would view me as a sloth who seeks any excuse to avoid showing up for work. Because of that worry, I'm writing under an assumed name.

Unfortunately, I can't say that ADD isn't a trendy label for attention deficit hyperactivity disorder. However, my treatment was so relieving that I no longer give a damn.

CHAPTER 11. SETTING UP YOURSELF FOR SUCCESS

Some jobs may be challenging for people with ADHD, especially if they don't interest them. If you're an adult with ADHD, your best bet for professional success is to find a line of work that requires both physical and mental activity. You'll need to make changes even in a fascinating field.

Dealing With Problems And Distractions

Get an evaluation done. Diagnosing ADHD requires a medical evaluation. Permit a trained professional to assess your work habits and suggest how you might grow. Taking this evaluation will help you identify your areas of strength and growth, allowing you to make the necessary adjustments to your approach to work.

Because a therapist or career counselor has the training and experience you lack, they can provide valuable insight that you might be missing without an outside perspective. In response, you can take steps to improve your situation.

1 Reduce outside distractions. Distractions and stressors can harm your productivity. You might be able to get more done if you eliminate these distractions. You may need to coordinate with your manager to minimize distractions.

- Reducing the number of people around you in the workplace is one approach to getting more work done without distraction. If you normally have trouble getting started on time, you could discover that arriving early helps you get more done.

- Close the door either figuratively or practically. Close the door to your office to avoid distractions. Avoid interruptions by working in a quiet area, such as a conference room, using white-noise headphones, or plugging your ears.

- Facing a wall and maintaining a clean workspace can also help reduce distractions.

2. Reduce internal distractions. It would help if you also addressed the internal distractions that stem from boredom and lack of imagination. Working against yourself can be just as counterproductive.

- Daydreaming is an example of an internal distraction. Idleness and procrastination are symptoms of excessive daydreaming. Perhaps you need to improvise some twists to spice things up a bit.

- It's also possible that thoughts will pop into your head unexpectedly. So always have a notepad handy to jot down any brilliant ideas.

- Additionally, you may become distracted if you suddenly realize that you need to get something done. Get a planner and a to-do list to help you reduce these.
- You could, for example, set a timer on your phone for every 30 minutes and spend a few minutes at that time being distracted.

3. Be mindful of the time. Hyperfocus has its benefits for productivity, but it can also lead to time management issues that hamper other endeavors. If you are daydreaming or losing track of time, try setting alerts on your phone or computer to snap you out of it.

4. Medications should be considered. Medication isn't the answer for everyone, but it could improve your performance at work. For example, taking medication for attention deficit hyperactivity disorder (ADHD) can improve concentration, leading to greater productivity and effectiveness. Find out if medicine could help you by consulting your doctor or a psychiatrist.

- Be sure to consult your doctor about the possibility of a once-daily drug covering you for the entire day. The timing of your commute to and from work could mean that a sleep aid that lasts eight hours won't be sufficient. An afternoon dose of a medication that lasts for four hours might be in order.

111

- Avoid using stimulant drugs late afternoon or evening if you want a good night's sleep. Instead, inform your doctor if you are having difficulties falling asleep.

Making Adjustments

1. Speak with your boss. Not every request can be met, but telling your manager how you function best at work will allow them to serve you better. They may be open to changing their management approach in return for your improved performance.

- People with attention deficit hyperactivity disorder (ADHD) benefit from, for instance, a combination of responsibility (such as a requirement to check in) and leeway (such as some leeway in how you manage your time).

- If you're having trouble keeping track of your tasks throughout the day, try asking your supervisor to create a thorough plan.

2. Always be ready to put forth extra effort if required. There will be moments as an adult with ADHD when you won't be able to meet all of your work's expectations because you'll be too distracted by other things. This necessitates extra effort to compensate for lost time and ensure you don't fall behind.

3. Get up and about whenever you can. Hyperactive people with ADHD should take every opportunity to get up and move around. For example, get up and walk around while you're talking on the phone or pay a visit to a coworker you've been meaning to talk to. You'll be more able to concentrate once you sit back down if you get up and move around first.

- Other similar changes may also help. For example, you might prefer to work while standing up or find that having "fidget" toys handy helps you concentrate better.

4. Put your hyperfocus to good use. Adults with ADHD often exhibit a laser-like focus when engaged in something they care deeply about. In the office, that's a huge plus because it means you can do much more in less time if you enjoy your profession.

- As a result, you'll be able to outperform your coworkers and earn your boss's praise by completing more tasks in less time. To that end, showing enthusiasm for your work will make your manager more likely to assign you new responsibilities.
-

Career And Field Selection

1. Select an active profession. To thrive as an adult with ADHD, it can help to pursue a line of work that requires moderate physical activity. As a person with ADHD, you probably wouldn't be happy sitting behind a desk all day. Consider fields of work that will keep you energized throughout the day if you want to increase your chances of success.

- Not all people who are "active" engage in strenuous physical activity. Mentally stimulating and challenging work can be beneficial in the same ways that physical work does.

- As adults, those with ADHD can find success in a variety of occupations, including show business, sales, politics, and emergency medical.

2. Examine many areas of interest. It's crucial to research before making a drastic professional change, whether you're just starting out or in the middle of your career. If you're already in the middle of your career, switching fields may prove just as challenging as your current job. However, as a newcomer, you should focus on building a bright future for yourself.

- Conduct research in your new field. Learn more about the job's requirements by looking it up online.

- Don't limit your research to the internet, though. Instead, contact a professional in the industry to learn more about typical tasks and responsibilities. Asking to work under someone else's supervision is another option for exploring whether or not the field is right for you.

3. Look for a job where your skills and interests are appreciated. You should choose an active job within a field that may or may not be active. Consider transitioning to a professional field you find interesting, if at all possible. Most career sectors feature both less active and more active positions.

- If your current position requires you to deal solely with paperwork, you might find more fulfillment in a role that involves more interaction with clients or customers.

CHAPTER 12. LOVING YOURSELF

Valentine's Day often brings up the idea that love is mysterious. Nevertheless, some people look forward to this day all year since it is their time to show appreciation to or get appreciation from the people they care about.

Insecurities, rejection, and low self-esteem can prevent adults with ADHD from fully appreciating the love they get from others and giving themselves.

What Is Self-esteem?

Self-esteem refers to how you perceive yourself. It's your honest assessment of your capabilities and limitations. Humans with a robust sense of self-worth know how to celebrate their achievements and simultaneously have compassion for their flaws. They have high standards for themselves and demand the same from others.

Is There A Link Between ADHD And Low Self-esteem?

Negative experiences and outcomes are common for people with ADHD because of the disorder's hallmark symptoms, which include poor focus, forgetfulness, and an obsession with instant satisfaction.

How To Improve Your Self-Esteem If You Have ADHD

You can do many things, and the best part is that you are in charge of them all, which will help boost your self-esteem. In addition, you can do anything on your own without anyone's help.

- **Believe In Yourself**

Having your confidence shaken by failure after failure is a certain way to lower your self-worth. You start to question your skills and abilities as a result of this. Believing in yourself is a great first step toward breaking the cycle and improving your self-esteem. While it may be trite to say, "Just believe in yourself," doing so is a crucial first step in building confidence.

- **Forget The Past**

You need a new beginning! Someone or something has made life difficult, if not impossible, for each of us at some point. So don't shut the door on a good future just because of a bad present or someone else's insecurity or lack of understanding.

Admit that you've been affected by the emotions and circumstances that led you here, but resolve to go on. Make up your mind that you will not let past wounds and regrets affect your present and future.

- **Learn To Forgive Yourself**

Surely by now, you have already served your punishment for your past transgressions. It would help if you stopped torturing and beating yourself over this blunder. This behavior serves no useful purpose for you or anybody else and is holding you back from reaching your full potential. Look instead for the lessons that can be drawn from this event. We can only take the lessons we've learned and resolve not to repeat our errors if we make them. ...let it go.

- **What's The Old Adage? "If you can't say anything pleasant, don't say anything at all."**

The adage "If you can't say anything pleasant, don't say anything at all" is one that most of us have internalized. Think of yourself as included in this. To this day, many of us keep on putting ourselves down, either out loud or internally.

Put an end to your negative self-talk and the destructive cycle of self-doubt that keeps replaying in your mind.

There is a part of each of us that acts as an inner critic or "gremlin," constantly questioning our self-confidence with statements like, "How could you be so stupid?"

- "No matter what you do, it turns out wrong."
- "Put another way: "Who do you think you are?"
- "You'll never master this, so give up now."

Rather, remind your inner critic, "If you can't say anything pleasant..." to lessen the impact of these unfavorable ideas.

- **Focus On Your Strengths**

The abilities and skills that come naturally to each of us set us apart. Your thoughts? If unsure, try keeping track of the things you find simple over the next week. For example, in what ways do you take pride in your accomplishments, and how do they make you feel when others praise you for them? There are hints everywhere!

Taking the time to reflect on such details is a surefire method of boosting your confidence. Spend most of your time doing what you're already good at rather than striving to improve at challenging things. You can apply this idea to your work, relationships, and free time.

- **It's Time To Take Action**

Make it a daily habit to work on your long-term goals. No matter how modest, taking action in the right direction will help you progress. On those days, it may be as simple as compiling a list of your five best qualities.

Other days may include devoting more time and energy to carrying out the tasks on your "to-do" list or developing a more comprehensive strategy to realize your goal. You can achieve your goals if you take methodical baby steps.

- **Sharpen Your Skills**

In addition to honing in on what you do well, becoming successful and having a healthy sense of self-worth requires mastering a few fundamentals. For someone with ADHD, these abilities may not come easily. One can, however, learn to master them over time.

Master the skills necessary to become a true professional:

- **Time Manager**: Being punctual gives the impression that you can be counted on.

- **Money Manager**: Neglecting to pay your mortgage or other large bills can seriously blow your pride.

- **Meal Planner**: You won't be at your best when you're hungry or snacking on junk food.

- **Housekeeper**: Having a messy, odorous home can seriously damage your self-esteem.

Due to the skills requirements, you may find certain jobs more difficult to complete because of your ADHD. However, mastery of each is not impossible.

- **Give Yourself A Compliment**

How you were complimented and corrected as a kid shapes your feelings. Adverse comments are sometimes made about children with ADHD rather than compliments. If you're like many adults, you've probably spent a lot of time dwelling on the things you've done "wrong" or aren't proud of.

Instead of being so hard on yourself, try to find two positives for every negative. Your sense of well-being will increase due to this redressing of the scales.

- **Avoid Making Unfair Comparisons To Others**

The practice of comparing yourself to others is common among children. Perhaps some of your friends and siblings found it easier to pay attention in class or remain seated than it was for you. But unfortunately, the tendency to compare oneself unfavorably with others harms self-esteem because we hardly ever do the opposite.

- **Laugh It Up!**

Get loud with your laughter. You can get people curious about your whereabouts by expressing pleasantly. Do it barefoot. Do whatever makes you laugh out loud or smile widely.

Everything about you, your life, your relationships, and your surroundings was created for pleasure. Too much magic and wonder await us here on Earth for us to waste any of it in apathy. Invest time in what makes you happy.

- **Keep It Real**

Amazing, natural talents abound in people with ADHD but are rarely fostered or recognized. So you should not be surprised at your lack of self-esteem. As a people, we have spent far too much time fooling ourselves into thinking that we are more capable than we are.

Just be yourself and stop pretending! Your skills and abilities are one-of-a-kind and should be shared with the world. If you've spent your life conforming to other people's expectations, you should know it's time to give up that effort.

Let go of the past, forgive yourself, take action, enjoy life, and be authentic; the loving life you deserve is within your reach.

CONCLUSION

A hasty diagnosis of attention deficit hyperactivity disorder (ADHD) in kids is too common. Symptoms are typically easy to identify and respond to treatment for. But if it isn't caught early, ADHD can cause serious issues in adulthood. At any point from adolescence to adulthood, this issue could resurface.

The NIMH estimates that 4 percent of adults have ADHD. Children with this disorder generally have trouble paying attention, can't control their impulses, and have explosive fits of energy.

However, adult symptoms are not always obvious and can lead to many problems if left untreated. However, identifying if you have ADHD might be difficult.

- Brain injuries.
- Exposure at an early childhood to harmful substances in the environment or in vitro.
- Use of alcoholic drinks and tobacco during pregnancy.
- Premature birth deliveries.
- Low birth weight.

There is still a lot of mystery around what causes ADHD, but contrary to popular belief, it is not related to things like food or family dynamics.

Which Symptoms Of Adult ADHD Are The Most Telling?

Adults are more challenging to diagnose than children; thus, neuropsychologists search for various signs when assessing adults for ADHD. Subtle indicators that show in daily activities are common among adult males. If you suspect you have adult ADHD, look at the following list of signs and symptoms.

- Neither your physical possessions nor your mental state can stay in any order.
- You pose a greater risk of causing collisions due to your increased tendency to drive at unsafe speeds.
- You have problems paying attention and listening.
- You have a hard time starting and keeping relationships.
- Typically, you're a restless person.
- You have a penchant for putting things off until the last possible minute.
- I feel bothered when you are late.

- Your emotions are overwhelming you.
- As a young child, you struggled through school.

In many ways, these issues in men as adults are only an evolution of problems faced by boys and men as youngsters. The body has adjusted to these routines since the illness has been untreated for so long.

Signs Of ADHD That Are Less Common In Males

Adult males with ADHD often have symptoms that amplify those seen in younger boys. In addition, these symptoms are often associated with an ADHD diagnosis, so it's more likely that a professional will notice them and make a diagnosis. Some of the less common symptoms of ADHD in adult males may include, though:

The use of frequent restroom breaks. Adult ADHD can also appear in less conventional ways, such as frequent restroom visits. You don't have to, but going would satisfy your body's exercise needs. People's impulse to move around is suppressed when they sit for long periods, such as during meetings or movies. It forces you to get up and go to the bathroom or get water more frequently.

Interrupting everyone all the time. If you're having a trying conversation with someone, and it seems like forever until they finish a sentence, you might be tempted to complete it for them. Perhaps you have a habit of interjecting your ideas into theirs. This behavior may have more to do with memory than simple impatience, and many adult males with ADHD may exhibit it. You might lose your communication ability if you don't say what's on your mind.

A passion for beginning new hobbies. Do you always want to find something that will pique your interest? Do you try to occupy your time with gaming, sports, or hobbies? A need for constant stimulation characterizes adult male ADHD. The problem is that few people stick with their newfound hobby.

Being glued to one's phone at all times. ADHD-afflicted adult men have trouble focusing on one thing at a time. As a result, they're looking to fill a hole in their lives, and relying heavily on their phones is a simple and convenient option. Males with ADHD might take a break from monotonous activities by talking on the phone. Any sense of anticipation is likewise diminished.

How Do Doctors Diagnose Adult ADHD?

If any of these symptoms sound familiar and you're worried about how they might affect your quality of life, it's time to make an appointment with your doctor. Your doctor will examine you and your symptoms to understand better what's going on with you. As a result, you must do the following:

- It's important to get checked out to make sure there's nothing else going on with your health.

- Please provide information on the duration of your symptoms, their onset, and other relevant medical background information.

- To further evaluate your symptoms, you should take a psychological test and the ADHD rating scales.

By taking these procedures, you and your doctor will have more information to assess your condition and choose future steps. You or your child's attention deficit hyperactivity disorder treatment will depend on this.

What Does Treatment Look Like?
Several medicines are available for the treatment and management of adult ADHD. Possible alternatives include:

- **Stimulants such as methylphenidate or amphetamine**. This helps keep your mental state steady and balanced. In addition, it ensures the proper functioning of your neurotransmitters.

- **Atomoxetine and bupropion are examples of non-stimulant drugs**. Taking these antidepressants may assist if you've experienced depression due to taking stimulants and are now looking for a more peaceful solution.

Naturally, you and your doctor need to talk about the treatment plan. Your doctor is the best person to address your worries and inquiries. Behavioral therapists can also help treat ADHD by teaching patients new skills for managing their feelings and focusing their energy.

Made in the USA
Monee, IL
12 June 2023

35635121R00070